Bra

pregnancy: how to enjoy it

gurgle
.com

pregnancy: how to enjoy it

Collins

First published in 2009 by
Collins, an imprint of
HarperCollins Publishers
77-85 Fulham Palace Road
London W6 8JB
www.collins.co.uk

Collins is a registered trademark of HarperCollins Publishers Ltd

Project Editor: Corinne Roberts
Design: Heike Schüssler and Cooling Brown
Cover Design: Heike Schüssler

ISBN: 978 0 00 728918 9

Colour reproduction by Dot Gradations, Essex
Printed and bound in Hong Kong by Printing Express

Contents

Foreword

The day after I gave birth to my first daughter, I was sitting in the maternity ward gazing adoringly at my tiny baby when the girl in the next bed, a second-time-around mum, leaned over and said, 'You should talk to your baby, you know, she'll love the sound of your voice and you haven't said anything to her yet. The more you speak to her, the quicker she'll learn to talk.' She was right. I was so busy admiring my new little bundle I hadn't uttered a word to her. I'd forgotten about my new role as her mum. From that moment on I plied the second-time-around-mum with the kind of questions I was too shy to ask the midwife: should my baby's legs be so curled up? Am I breastfeeding correctly? Are her fingers meant to be that purple and why am I so scared that something will happen to her if I go to the loo...

It was out of this constant need for answers that **gurgle.com** was born. I'm not the first mum who arrived home with a tiny baby feeling engulfed by the enormity of the task ahead. It didn't start there, the questions started before I became pregnant: what's ovulation? When will I fall pregnant? Will my morning sickness ever stop? At **gurgle.com** we try to provide parents and parents-to-be with a place they can visit for all those 3am worries, a place where they can see weekly updates of their child's development and above all a place where they can meet other parents going through exactly the same things they are. After all, having a baby is not a journey anyone should do alone.

The more we talked to the mums using **gurgle**, the more we realised that the same questions came up again and again. So we decided to publish a set of **gurgle** handbooks in response to the most asked questions on the site. We want these books to guide you through what mums have told us are the three trickiest areas of parenting: how to enjoy your pregnancy (and we promise you can), getting your baby into good sleep habits, and feeding your baby. We don't want to preach or tell you how it should be done, but we do want to provide you with lots of helpful information and tips based on the advice of both our **gurgle** panel of experts and our incredibly supportive and knowledgeable community of mums.

We want you to see our **gurgle** books as your older sister or best friend who has had a baby and is passing on her knowledge to you. We're the midwife who helps you with breastfeeding, or the auntie who suggests a way to help your baby sleep at night.

As much as I wanted to take my maternity ward 'neighbour' home with me, I couldn't. I had to learn how to become a parent, just as my daughter had to learn to sit, walk and talk. We hope that these books become that tap on the shoulder in the maternity ward giving you a friendly nudge in the right direction. Oh, and just for the record, my daughter is now a right little chatterbox...

Nifa McLaughlin
Editor of **gurgle.com** and mum to Ivy and Poppy

 We hope you enjoy our books and if we've missed anything out, please visit **gurgle.com** for lots more videos, groups, articles, chat and tools to complement these books. Register with **gurgle.com** and receive free weekly emails walking you through pregnancy and parenthood.

I'm pregnant – what next?

The big moment

Discovering you are pregnant is both an anxious yet exciting time, but after you have tested yourself and got that BFP ('big fat positive', to anyone not familiar with internet chatroom speak!), what next?

It's time to make an appointment with your GP. She probably won't do any additional pregnancy testing because home pregnancy tests are now so reliable (about 99.9% accurate). You'll need to tell her when the first day of your last period was and how many days your cycle usually lasts, and she will work out your due date. The average pregnancy lasts for 280 days or 40 weeks from the first day of your last period (although only 5% of babies stick to this date!). If you don't know the exact date of your last period, you are likely to be given a dating scan some time before 13 weeks.

Your GP will ask you which hospital you want to have your baby in. Most larger cities have two or more hospitals so take into consideration how close they are to your home and to your place of work as you may be attending antenatal appointments during working hours. Depending on your GP, she may or may not perform a blood test or ask for a sample of urine. If she doesn't, these tests will, in any case, be carried out at your first antenatal appointment. She may also measure your height and weigh you in order to monitor your weight gain in the forthcoming weeks.

Now is the chance to ask your GP any questions – for example, will you receive shared care in which half your antenatal appointments are at the maternity unit or clinic and half are at your doctor's surgery? If you still smoke or drink, or if you have taken drugs recently, you may want to tell your GP. From here, your GP will inform the hospital of your choice that you are pregnant and you will probably be contacted via the post with details of your first antenatal appointment.

 For the **gurgle** video on **Home pregnancy testing**, go to **gurgle.com** and click on **Videos**

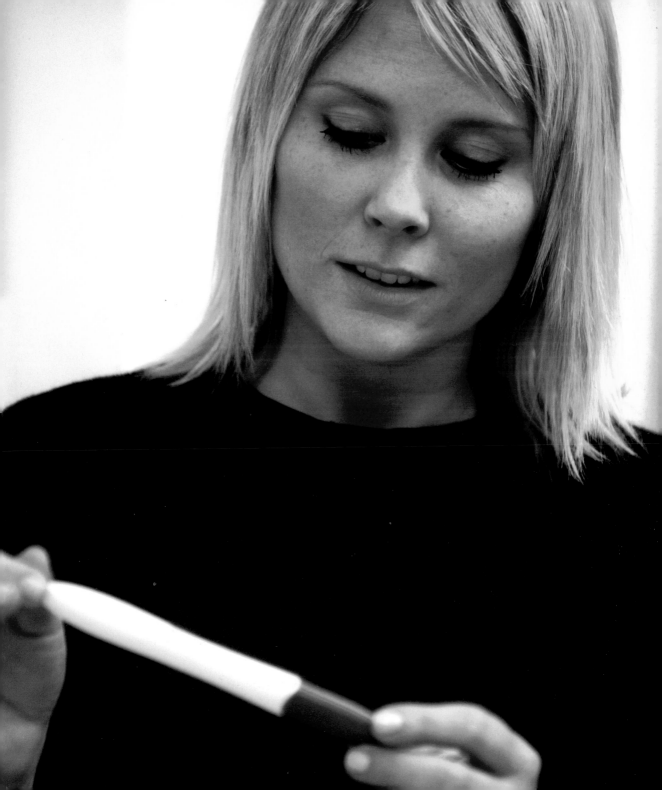

Your changing body

No two pregnancies are alike – just because your sister didn't have morning sickness doesn't mean you won't get it, unfortunately. Some women bloom while others have to put up with greasy hair and spots! Your own pregnancy can vary from week to week and day to day.

In the first trimester (each trimester lasts three months), you will probably notice that, although you will still look pretty much the same, your body will begin to feel different physically, and you will also, no doubt, be going through significant changes mentally as you come to terms with your pregnancy. At around six weeks, you may start to feel very tired. Tiredness in pregnancy can feel a lot like jet lag – many women report getting home from work and wanting to go straight to bed. Not exactly ideal, but at least it doesn't last for the whole nine months. The tiredness is thought to be due to rising levels of pregnancy hormones in your body. These will be busy forming the placenta, your baby's support system, which takes over at around 12–14 weeks.

Morning sickness, or pregnancy sickness (renamed because it is not just confined to the morning), may appear soon after the feelings of

Mum's top tip

I was a bag of tears in the early weeks of my third pregnancy, but now, in week 14, I'm so much more energetic and I've stopped feeling sick. Just remember that what you experience with one pregnancy doesn't mean the others will be the same. Every woman is different and so is her growing bump and changing body. Your body is going through an enormous change right now. Don't be too hard on yourself. Have a bath, paint your nails, grab a coffee with a friend. Take things easy!

I'm pregnant – what next?

fatigue have abated. While some women don't suffer from morning sickness, most don't escape it, unfortunately. The sickness, or feelings of nausea, are again down to the rapid rise within your body of oestrogen and the pregnancy hormone human chorionic gonadotrophin (HCG). During pregnancy your sense of smell is also heightened, making you gag at things that would never have troubled you before – the smell of coffee, a friend's perfume or a cigarette.

In early pregnancy you will find that some days you feel fine and full of energy while at other times you'll be longing for a nap by 3pm! Unfortunately, you may not have let on to other people just yet, early pregnancy being when most women keep their pregnancies a secret until they get to around 12 weeks when the chances of miscarriage decrease dramatically.

It isn't just you going through immense changes, your baby is growing rapidly too. He has changed from being just a cluster of cells and is now forming the rudimentary shape of a tiny foetus. His heart will have begun to form and will start beating around 22 days after conception. By the fifth week, he will be about 1.25mm ($^1/_{20}$in) long and his brain, spinal cord, nervous system and throat will have begun to develop.

Even though your baby's development slows down during the second and third trimesters, when he is fully formed, he still needs to put on lots of weight and grow. Somewhere between 18 and 20 weeks, you may feel him kicking for the first time. Your baby will spend much of the second trimester and most of the third exploring his senses, especially touch and taste. In the third trimester, he will spend most of his time concentrating on getting bigger and preparing for life outside the womb. His lungs will be the last organ to develop fully, because he doesn't need them for breathing until he's outside the womb. This is why many premature babies need help breathing when they are first born.

Pregnancy week by week

ONE TO THREE WEEKS

Congratulations! It's now that your amazing journey of becoming a mother really begins. For the first month most women don't even know they are pregnant, but huge changes are happening in your body, even though the physical signs won't reveal themselves for some time. Folic acid plays a large role in cell growth and development as well as in tissue formation. Are you remembering to take supplements? (See page 42.)

This early stage of pregnancy is extremely important because your baby, a fraction of a millimetre at this point, is changing from a cluster of cells to form a tiny embryo. Even though it's far too early to tell, your baby's sex has already been decided at the point of conception, as well as all the distinguishing features such as eye and hair colour, height and foot size. You will have to wait a little longer to find out the sex, though...

FOUR WEEKS

By this week, your fertilized egg has embedded into the delicate lining of your uterus and the mass of cells which will eventually become your baby continues to divide and multiply. Even though miraculous events are taking place and a new life is starting to form, your baby is still only about 1mm ($\frac{1}{25}$in) long. Week four is usually regarded as the beginning of the embryonic period as your baby's major organs and spine all start to develop from now on. At around 22 days a primitive heart has already begun to beat. This means absolutely no alcohol or smoking as both can cause damage to the foetus.

FIVE WEEKS

If you can smell the perfume of someone on the other side of the office, or you suddenly go off your favourite chai tea latte, it's just one of many peculiar quirks of pregnancy. You may need to nip to the loo more frequently because your uterus is constantly enlarging (from plum-sized before pregnancy to melon-sized at 40 weeks) and pressing on your bladder, forcing you to make many a midnight dash.

Your baby is now about 1.25mm ($\frac{1}{20}$in) long and has lost the little tail she had when she first developed. She now looks a lot more like a baby and even does jumpy movements from time to time. You won't feel her moving for a while, but the physical changes your body is going through will remind you constantly that you are pregnant.

SIX WEEKS

This week your baby has almost doubled in size to some-where between 2 and 4mm ($\frac{1}{15}$ and $\frac{1}{5}$in). If you could look inside yourself, you would see a huge head in proportion to her body as the head grows faster to accommodate the growing brain. Your baby's eyes and ears are also beginning to form, as well as four tiny buds on the centre of her body that will eventually become her arms and legs.

Some women don't feel pregnant at this stage, while others will be subjected to the 'pleasures' of pregnancy, such as so-called morning sickness but which seems to go on all day (and half the night), extreme tiredness and needing the loo more often. These can all be tricky to explain if nobody at work knows you are pregnant. Try to rest as much as possible when you're at home and consider telling one trusted colleague you are pregnant, so that they can help make excuses when everybody goes for after-work drinks.

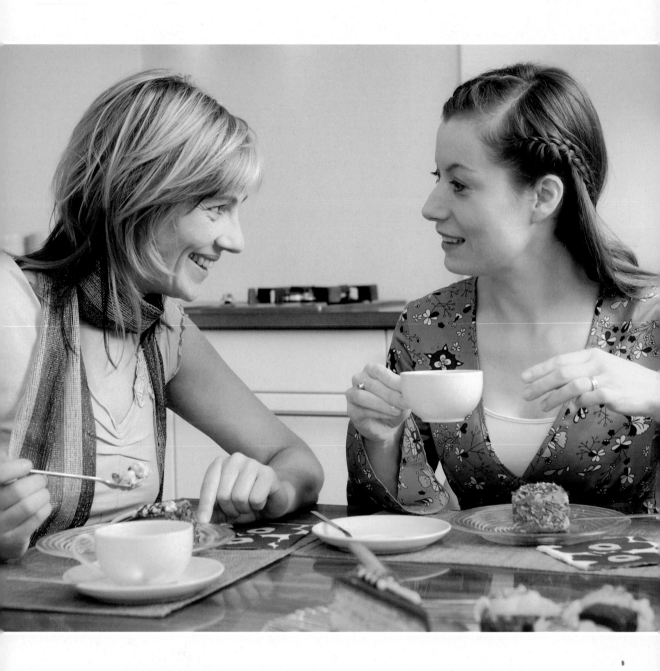

I'm pregnant – what next?

SEVEN WEEKS

Your baby's facial features are starting to develop this week, with tiny nostrils and eyelids forming, as well as pigmentation in the irises of the eyes. Your baby is now about the size of a kidney bean and is continuing to grow at an astonishing rate. Although still minute, she is starting to resemble a tiny human being at this stage.

All babies are potentially at some risk of developing spina bifida and other neural tube defects that affect the development of the brain and spinal cord. Most of these defects occur in the early stages of pregnancy, which is why it's vital to start taking folic acid before you're pregnant and throughout the first trimester.

EIGHT WEEKS

This week, depending on whether your baby is a boy or a girl, the gonads (the primary reproductive organs) become either ovaries or testes. Although the sex of your child was decided weeks ago, at the point of conception, it is still too early to tell what sex your baby will be using an ultrasound scan.

If you could see your baby now, you would observe a tiny nose beginning to form, as well as the jaw, which will eventually become her mouth.

Your baby is beginning to move around this week, in jumpy little movements, but she is still too small for you to be able to feel her move at this stage.

NINE WEEKS

This week your baby has grown to about the size of a grape (about 2–3cm/^{3}/$_4$-1in long). His back is straightening, his neck is becoming more erect and his eyes are now fully developed, although they won't open for some time. Webbed fingers and toes are developing on the tiny buds that will become his arms and legs. Don't worry: your baby will lose the webbed appearance before birth – he isn't turning into a frog!

Physically, you could be feeling particularly tired this week. You may notice your breasts beginning to swell and your nipples turning a shade darker. These are all normal signs of being pregnant.

TEN WEEKS

This is a landmark week in your pregnancy because your baby's internal organs, including his heart, are completely formed and fully functional. Now all they need to do is get bigger, along with the rest of your baby. This week tiny tooth buds are forming in his mouth that will become his milk teeth some time in his first year. Your baby's senses are developing, too: for the first time, he will be able to taste the amniotic fluid he is swallowing.

For you, morning sickness tends to be worse around this time, when the pregnancy hormone HCG reaches a peak. But don't worry – for most women nausea starts to ease off from now onwards and usually disappears by week 12. Because of hormonal changes, some women break out in spots, but this should settle down after week 12, when hormonal activity will have levelled out a bit.

11 WEEKS

You are now almost at the second trimester, when the incidence of miscarriage decreases dramatically and it will feel safer to reveal to everyone why you have been so grumpy and tired lately, and spending so much time in the bathroom. Your baby is now about the size of a large lime and is busy kicking and stretching inside you. You won't feel any flutterings until he gets bigger, but if you could look inside, you would see your baby doing tiny hiccups as his diaphragm practises working. Over the next few weeks, he will increase in size and almost double in length. During pregnancy the higher levels of oestrogen flowing around your body mean that your hair is less likely to shed and may be thicker and shinier than it was pre-pregnancy. Unfortunately, your body hair may be flourishing rather more too, so don't be surprised if you are constantly having to shave!

12 WEEKS

At 12 weeks, you may notice some of the less welcome elements of early pregnancy – morning sickness and extreme tiredness – starting to subside. Your baby's development has passed the critical stage this week and there'll be less chance of you miscarrying from now on. You may want to start telling people you are pregnant – unless you've told the world already! This week your baby is beginning to practise using his reflexes. If his hands or feet touch any other part of his body, he may flinch, and if they brush his eyes, he may blink in response. If you prod your uterus, your baby will squirm away, but he is still too small for you to feel anything yet. If your stomach looks bloated, it won't be because of your baby but because of the pregnancy hormones slowing down your bowels and digestive system.

13 WEEKS

By week 13, the beginning of the second trimester, many women notice that morning sickness tends to have subsided. Instead of feeling exhausted, you may begin to get your normal energy levels back and actually start enjoying the fact that you are pregnant.

This week your baby measures between 6.5–8cm (2$\frac{1}{2}$– 3$\frac{1}{4}$in) in length and is busy sucking (getting herself ready for breastfeeding), swallowing and wriggling about. She is also starting to look increasingly like a tiny human being as her head and neck move up and become straighter, and less like a little prawn.

14 WEEKS

This week your baby will be practising lots of new skills; her digestive system will be starting to move food through her body, and she will be busy weeing into the amniotic fluid. She will also be breathing in amniotic fluid to and from her lungs, to prepare her for breathing properly once she is born. Eyelids, fingernails and toenails are developing rapidly and tiny hairs are growing all over her body.

By week 14, your hormones will be steadying as your baby's placenta takes over supporting her, giving your body a welcome rest! There's no rest for your tummy, though; from now on, you may be able to see a little bump appearing, as your uterus continues to move further up your abdomen, occupying the area from just below your pubic line to your navel. Although it's early days yet, maternity trousers or something not too tightly fitting around your stomach might help you feel more comfortable.

15 WEEKS

At week 15, your baby will be practising gestures that make her appear more and more human. She can yawn, blink and rub her eyes, and she carries on wriggling around, kicking her legs and waving her arms. The hair on her head is beginning to grow and the hairline she will have when she is born now starts to form.

As your uterus grows and your belly starts to expand, you may acquire stretch marks as your skin stretches to accommodate your baby. Unfortunately there is not much you can do to stop these occurring, but rubbing olive oil on your lower abdomen twice a day may help to keep the skin supple and moisturized.

16 WEEKS

This week your baby has grown to about the size of an avocado. If you could see inside, you might see her wiggling her fingers and toes as she practises coordinating her limbs. Her circulatory system is in proper working order, while her urinary tract has matured enough to enable her to have a wee every 40 minutes.

Her arms and legs are now fully formed and throughout her body bones are starting to ossify (harden). This week your baby is very active, but if this is your first baby you probably won't feel her moving for a few weeks yet. If you have already had a baby, you may recognize the familiar fluttering feeling in your tummy, however, as your baby wriggles and somersaults in your womb.

17 WEEKS

At week 17, your baby would now fit into the palm of your hand. Fatty deposits are starting to be laid down under the skin ready to help your baby maintain her body temperature once she is born. Connections are forming all the time between her brain, muscles and nervous system, and her tiny heart is busy pumping about 25 litres (42 pints) of blood around her body every day!

You may start to notice considerable changes in your breasts this week. They may acquire a more veiny appearance as well as increasing by one cup size. The areola, or skin around each nipple, and your nipples themselves will start to get darker, as well as increasing in size. A line may appear from your belly button down your navel. This line, known as the *linea nigra*, will continue to darken throughout your pregnancy, then vanish once you have had your baby.

18 WEEKS

Feeling any movement yet? Don't worry if you're not – lots of women don't feel their babies move until 20–24 weeks – but expect to feel it very soon. This week your ligaments are getting softer as your pelvis prepares to widen in preparation for the birth. Be careful not to over-exert yourself, and make sure you stick to gentle exercises at this time, rather than anything too strenuous.

Meanwhile, your baby's immune system is starting to mature in preparation for life outside the womb and her intestines are beginning to collect meconium – ready for her first poo! As well as being able to stretch out all parts of her body, your baby can now rotate her head and move her tongue.

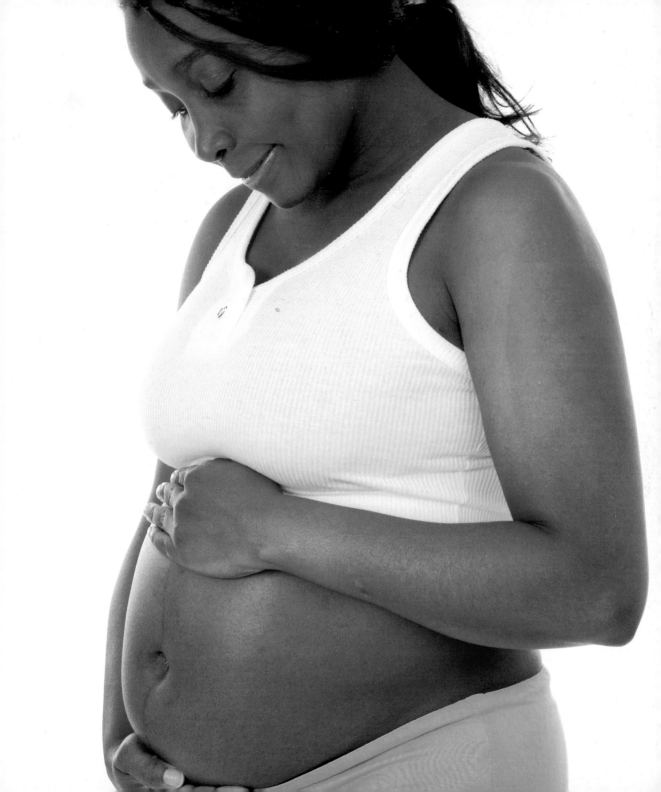

19 WEEKS

Your bump is really starting to show this week and you may feel a fluttering sensation inside as your baby practises kicks and somersaults. At week 19, he's now big enough for you to feel him move. It is also about now that a few pregnancy aches and pains may start to happen as your body copes with the extra weight of your growing bump.

If you were able to look inside your body, you would see that your baby is now covered by a protective coating of a waxy white substance called vernix, while his legs and arms have reached a size where they are now in the right proportion to his body. If you are carrying a girl, her ovaries now have around 6 million eggs, a number that will reduce to 2 million by the time he is born.

20 WEEKS

Congratulations – you are halfway through your pregnancy! For some women, 20 weeks of pregancy will have seemed like an eternity, while for others it will have flown by (probably those who didn't suffer from morning sickness!). It is only another 20 weeks (give or take a couple) until you meet your baby! By 18–20 weeks, you will have a routine ultrasound or foetal anomaly scan that can identify the sex of your baby and check that he has reached the right size for the stage of pregnancy.

Before you get too excited about discovering the sex of your baby, it is worth bearing in mind that sometimes this cannot be verified as your baby may be turning away during the scan or crossing his legs. Equally, if you don't want to know the sex of your baby at this stage, it's a good idea to tell the sonographer in case you get an accidental glimpse!

21 WEEKS

This week (for most women, anyway) it's officially goodbye to your waistline. Some women love the look of their swollen, pregnant bellies, but don't worry if you aren't among them and regard your changing figure with dismay. Most women go through a stage where they long to have their pre-pregnancy figure back.

This week your baby is roughly the same length as a banana (about 16cm/6$\frac{1}{3}$in), half the size he'll be when he's born. Although his growth rate has slowed down, his heartbeat is getting stronger every day and his hearing is improving. Your baby will be able to hear as soon as he is born and may turn towards your voice when he hears you speak, recognizing it from when he heard it in the womb. So make sure you talk as much as possible to your growing bump!

22 WEEKS

Your baby's facial features are now very well developed. If you could see him, you would make out tiny closed eyes (his eyelids are still fused together), a minute button nose and mouth, eyelashes, eyebrows and even hair on his head. From now on, your baby's movements are very deliberate as he stretches his limbs, sucks his thumb and hiccups (which you may feel). Practising these movements will help him to improve his coordination and fine motor skills once he is born.

As your body continues to grow, you may experience some weight gain, but don't let this be an excuse to eat badly or take no exercise. Gentle swimming, pregnancy yoga or taking a short walk can help you to stay fit. (See pages 56–9 for more information.)

23 WEEKS

In this middle stage of pregnancy, when your bump isn't huge and you feel energized and full of beans, it might be a good idea to go away on holiday or for a long weekend. Very soon you won't be able to have spontaneous nights out with your partner, or weekends away, without sore boobs and a crying baby. You can fly while pregnant until your 34th week, so why not book somewhere decadent while you can?

Now that you can feel your baby kicking, you may start to notice a cycle of times when he is asleep and times when he's awake and active. This week the hair on your baby's head begins to darken to the colour it will be when he is born.

24 WEEKS

Week 24 is an exciting milestone to have reached because from now on your baby will have a chance of surviving outside the womb if he arrives early. His hearing is developing all the time and he can now detect sounds outside the uterus as well as inside your body. He can hear your voice too, so talk to him as much as you can.

This week you may notice you keep knocking things over, stubbing your toes or wobbling slightly as you walk. The reason for this is that your centre of gravity has changed because your uterus, baby and therefore most of your weight is focused in the middle of your body.

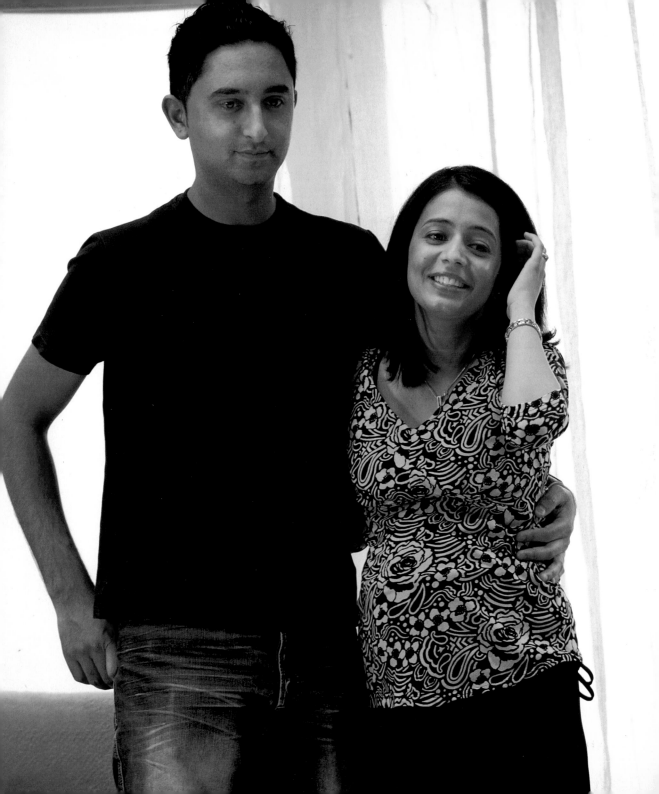

25 WEEKS

This week your baby's dexterity starts to improve, which means she can curl her fingers into a fist or grab the umbilical cord. In her gums her adult teeth are starting to form, but won't appear until her milk teeth fall out at around age six. By 25 weeks, your baby's brainwave patterns are similar to what they will be when she is born, which means she is already acquiring a primitive memory. Keep singing and talking to your baby because she will become familiar with your voice and the songs you sing to her in the womb. You may start to feel breathless this week as your uterus moves into your ribcage and presses against your lungs.

26 WEEKS

This week you may notice your baby becoming very active, particularly after you have eaten. The best thing about being able to feel your baby kick is that you can monitor her on a daily basis and be reassured by every move, although some babies are more active than others in the womb. Fat is continuing to form under your baby's skin – essential for keeping her warm after she is born. Newborn babies find it hard to regulate their body temperatures, however, which is why the maternity ward is always so hot!

At week 26, your baby is about 23cm (9in) in length and studies show she can now respond to touch. If you prod your lower abdomen, you may feel her squirming away and at your antenatal checks when the midwife feels your stomach, you may notice your baby kicking to get away! You may find you feel heavier by the afternoon when you are more bloated as your body is retaining more water, so if you can, make sure you sit down more or have an afternoon nap. This week may be when you say goodbye to seeing your toes for a while!

27 WEEKS

Congratulations – you have made it to the third trimester! From now on, your baby will continue to put on fat and grow and your tummy will reach magnificent proportions! From now until 30 weeks, your baby goes through a very active phase as she attempts to somersault and kick in an increasingly cramped environment. This, combined with a decrease in the amount of amniotic fluid surrounding your baby, accounts for why you now feel that every blow is aimed at your bladder!

Look out for signs of pre-eclampsia from this point onwards. If your hands, feet and face suddenly swell, you have high blood pressure and there is protein in your urine (which will be spotted at antenatal checks), consult your doctor or midwife straight away to rule out anything serious. (For more on pre-eclampsia, see page 102–3.)

28 WEEKS

Your baby's eyes are beginning to open this week and if she touches her eyes with her fingers, her immediate reaction is to blink. Meconium (your baby's first poo) continues to be formed in her intestines, ready to come out a short while after birth. If your baby were to be born now, she would have a 95% chance of survival, with medical assistance. If you are having a boy, his testes will be descending from his abdomen to his groin about now.

You may experience pressure on your bladder this week, as your uterus grows bigger and impacts on everything that surrounds it. Just like your first trimester, you may need to make those midnight dashes to the toilet once again.

29 WEEKS

Most of your baby's development from now on concerns maturing in preparation for life outside his watery world. Your baby's eye colour is now a slate grey/blue and he is opening his eyes from time to time. Blood vessels are maturing in his lungs, so that when he is born he will be ready to take his first breath. If you could look at your baby now, you would see him practising his facial expressions!

By week 29, your stomach is probably feeling a bit squashed, so start eating frequent small meals rather than occasional large ones, and avoid dining late in the evening, when food is harder to digest. (For advice on eating healthily during pregnancy, see pages 42–7.)

30 WEEKS

It probably feels as if you've been pregnant for ever, especially when you look back to when you did your pregnancy test and discovered it was positive. Don't worry: there are only ten weeks to go (or thereabouts)! This week your baby measures around 27cm (10½in) and is able to recognize your voice. He's busy practising his breathing in preparation for when he has to use his lungs properly, although sometimes the amniotic fluid goes down the wrong way and makes him hiccup.

You may have already noticed your nipples becoming larger and much darker and your breasts looking more veiny in appearance. At this stage, some women may also notice a small amount of white substance leaking from their nipples. This is colostrum, the first milk your baby will drink if you plan to breastfeed.

31 WEEKS

Your baby is putting down more fat stores beneath his skin and gaining as much as 500g (17oz) a week. The hair that covers his skin, known as lanugo, is shedding slowly and will probably be gone by the time he's born. Although there isn't much room inside your uterus at the moment, your baby may move into a head-down position around this time – the ideal position for him to be born in.

Don't worry if you feel your baby moving less – it's not easy to somersault in an increasingly cramped environment. As long as you still feel him moving from time to time (usually after you eat), there is nothing to worry about.

32 WEEKS

By week 32, day-to-day tasks – such as bending to put your socks on or getting in and out of a car – are becoming increasingly difficult. As for painting your toenails, that's somewhere in the distant, non-pregnant past!

By this stage in pregnancy, your baby's five senses – touch, smell, taste, hearing and seeing – are all fully functioning and taking in the strange world he inhabits of the womb. Noises from your stomach gurgle close by, colours within the womb vary as the light outside changes the amount of light in the womb, and the comforting sound of your voice floats in to your baby.

You may notice your lower abdomen tightening occasionally from now onwards as your body practises Braxton Hicks contractions (see page 161) in preparation for the actual contractions of labour.

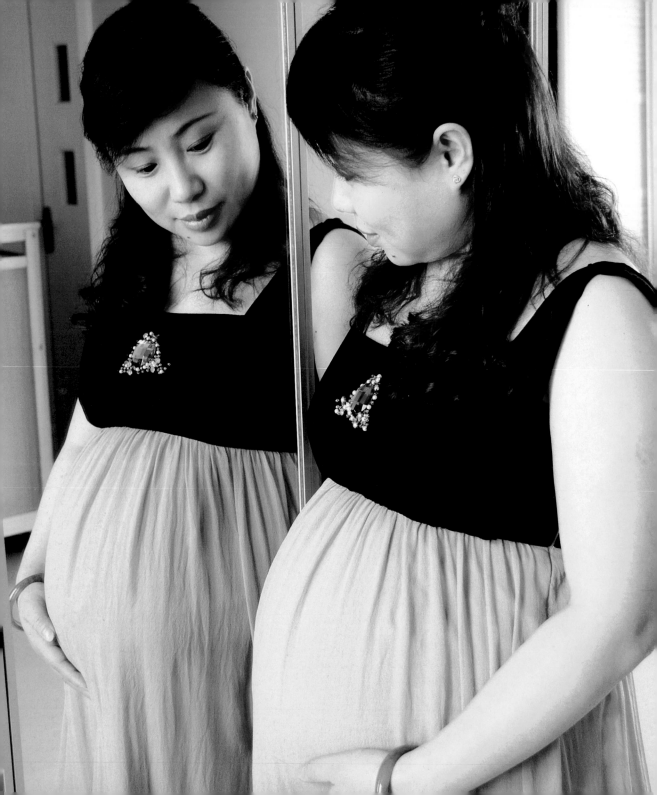

33 WEEKS

By week 33, it probably feels as if there is no room left inside you, and you would no doubt be glad if your baby popped out tonight! Even though he has a very good chance of surviving now if he were to arrive early, he may still have trouble breathing. It would be best for him to be born after 'term', which is 37 weeks. Not long to go, even so.

Your baby is about 30cm (11^3/$_4$in) long and he sleeps for most of the day and night, as it is too cramped in the womb for any somersaulting now. His skin has changed from reddish to bright pink. Dark-skinned babies may also have a reddish tinge, their skin remaining quite pale in the womb and after birth as the skin pigment melanin does not appear until some weeks or even months after the birth.

34 WEEKS

It is reassuring to know that if your baby were to be born now he would have a 95% chance of surviving – this time without medical assistance. The placenta reaches maturity at about this time and from here on it starts to age, its precious job of supporting your baby is nearly over.

At week 34, your baby is busy weeing (sometimes up to a 600ml/1 pint a day) into the amniotic fluid as his kidneys and digestive system are now fully functioning. If you are having a boy, his testicles may have ended their journey downwards into the scrotum by now.

If you shone a light at your stomach, your baby would be able to see it. At this point in his development, he can tell, from the amount of light in the womb, when you have moved from the muted light of a room to bright sunlight outdoors.

35 WEEKS

Sometime soon your cervix will begin to dilate in order to prepare for the birth of your baby. Some women experience a 'show', which is when the mucus plug at the top of the cervix dislodges as the cervix starts to dilate. Although it does not mean labour is going to start straight away, it is a sign that labour is imminent.

By now you will have become aware that your breasts are noticeably bigger, your nipples darker and the area around them (the areola) will have changed size. The *linea nigra* – the line running from your belly button down to your pubic region – is also darker. Don't worry, all these changes are unique to pregnancy, however, and will disappear once your baby is born.

36 WEEKS

You will probably start having antenatal checks about once a week from now until you give birth so you and your baby can be monitored for any problems such as pre-eclampsia (see pages 102–3). If she has started moving down the uterus or has already moved into a head-down position, you may feel a little respite in the pressure on your stomach and lungs. Breathing should be easier, and indigestion and heartburn less of a problem.

At week 36, your baby's fingernails are tiny but fully formed and very sharp. You may have to cut them as soon as she is born or invest in a pair of scratch gloves for her to wear. She still sleeps for about 90% of the time and this pattern will continue for a while after she is born.

37 WEEKS

Congratulations! You have reached full term, which means your baby may be born at any time. While you are considered to be full term at 37 weeks, you may not actually deliver until week 41 or later if this is your first baby. Don't worry; you'll meet your baby very soon!

If you could see your baby now, she would look like a newborn. She is plumper in appearance than she was a few weeks ago, but still covered in the creamy white substance called vernix. Her lungs are now fully developed and she would need no help to breathe if she were born now. People may remark that you have 'dropped', which means your baby has moved further down towards your pelvis in preparation for being born.

38 WEEKS

Keep reminding yourself 'the end is in sight' as you lug yourself around. This week can be particularly tiresome in hot weather. Despite this, you may have begun cleaning your house from top to bottom this week in a sudden burst of activity that is part of what is recognized as 'nesting' – getting everything ready for the arrival of your baby. It won't mean your baby is coming tonight, but labour may start in a week or so.

If you're worried about how your big 'bump' is going to fit down the birth canal, bear in mind that your baby's skull is designed to be soft and pliable in the womb, some bones not actually fusing together until after she is born. This should make it easier for her head to mould to the shape of the birth canal and vagina, which in turn will make the birth easier.

39 WEEKS

Now your feet have disappeared from view, you probably find yourself constantly bumping into things and stubbing your toes. Don't worry – very soon you will be able to see them again! You will probably have trouble performing simple tasks this week without huffing and puffing or having to sit down and rest every five minutes.

By week 39, your baby's digestive system has matured enough to be able to take liquid foods when she is born. If you haven't done so already, now is a good time to read up about breast- or bottlefeeding to prepare yourself for the coming months. Most of the hair that has covered and protected your baby's skin has fallen off. She probably weighs about 3kg (7lb) by now (although this is an average weight only) and continues to put down fat beneath her skin in preparation for life in the outside world

40 WEEKS

Although this week marks your official due date, not all mothers (especially first-timers) give birth precisely at this time. In fact most women give birth around two weeks before or two weeks after this date. At your antenatal appointment, you will be checked to make sure you and your baby are doing well.

Your baby probably measures around 37–38cm (14$\frac{1}{2}$–15in) in length and is completely ready to be born. If you feel her moving a lot less, don't worry; there is very little room for manoeuvre inside the cramped uterus. But as long as she still moves occasionally, there is nothing to worry about.

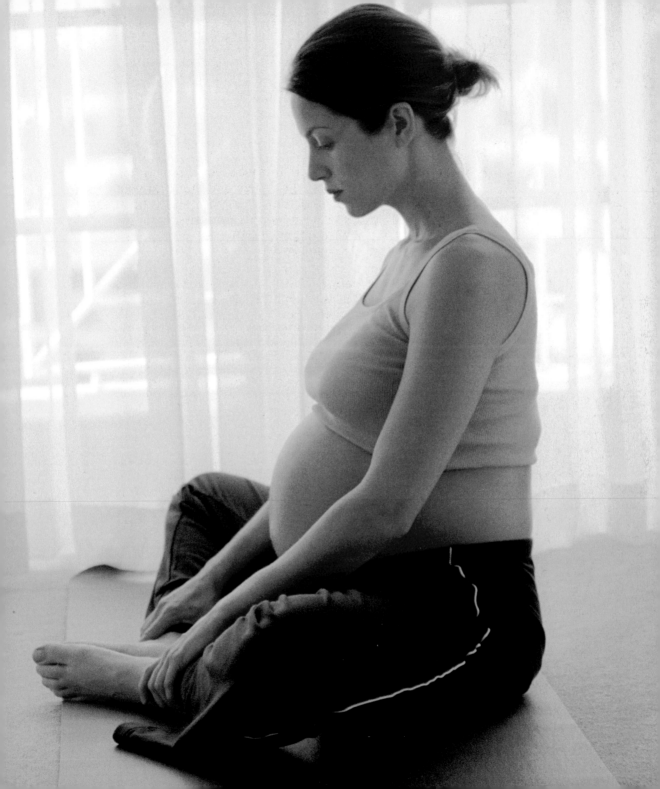

Dad-to-be: what to expect

As a dad-to-be, you're embarking on a journey with your partner that will end with the birth of your child and a new life for both of you. The journey to that point may not be an altogether smooth one, however. While you won't be carrying the baby yourself, you will be the one to whom your partner will look for comfort and support.

You may find it a testing time in your relationship as you support your partner through morning sickness, mood swings and the usual fears and worries that beset all mums-to-be. Getting ready for the arrival of your baby is an experience like no other, however, and the chances are you will come out of it stronger than ever, ready to face the exciting task of parenthood.

PREPARE WITH HER
When the time comes, get involved in buying things for your baby with your partner. Go to parentcraft classes together (see pages 110–11). This will give you a good opportunity to discuss your feelings and fears with other expectant parents, and with each other. If you can, accompany your partner to her antenatal scans and tests (see pages 86–9) so that you can see how your baby is developing in the womb. Seeing your baby moving on the screen will make it so much more real!

HELP HER COPE WITH THE SYMPTOMS OF PREGNANCY
Some women sail through pregnancy with a permanent bloom, while others experience the full brunt of morning sickness, cravings (see pages 54–5) and hormonal changes. In reality, most pregnancies have a bit of everything, good and bad. Your partner will be experiencing all sorts of new sensations, and she'll want to share these with you. Find out what you can do to be helpful, such as preparing snacks and drinks to help ease morning sickness, giving a back rub, or just being there to provide a sympathetic ear and a hug.

She may also experience emotional ups and downs during pregnancy (and beyond!), so don't be surprised if she becomes irritable and short-tempered. Try to be patient and calm with her and remember that this moodiness won't last, that it's all due to the rise in pregnancy hormones and the massive changes her body is undergoing during this time.

HELP HER TO BE HEALTHY
Giving up alcohol and certain foods is no fun for many women, so consider doing the same when you are together. If you are a smoker, this is definitely the time to quit. As your partner attempts to eat a healthy, balanced diet, try and do the same yourself. (For more information on healthy eating in pregnancy, see pages 42–7.)

DISCUSS YOUR FEELINGS ABOUT THE BIRTH
All mums-in-waiting have worries about the arrival of their baby. Will he be healthy? How will you both cope with the massive change in your lifestyle? You will probably share some of the same concerns; other worries may seem different but are in fact two sides of the same coin. For example, many men worry that their partner will be so bound up in the new baby that they will be pushed aside, while many women fear that their body will be less attractive to their partner after the birth, and that they might be rejected. Getting these issues out in the open before your baby is born, when it's possible to discuss such things more calmly and rationally, is better than letting them go unaddressed, only to erupt later and with greater force.

GIVE PRACTICAL SUPPORT DURING LABOUR
Read up on what happens during labour, and attend the antenatal classes that look specifically at what you can do to help as a dad. Your support during labour will be essential, so the more prepared you can be, the more help you will be to your partner. Familiarize yourself with the route to the hospital and make sure you know what you need to take with you.

Feeling good – yes, it's possible!

Diet for a healthy pregnancy

When you are pregnant, what you eat is of huge importance to the healthy development of your growing baby. Read on to find out which foods you need to include in your diet to make sure you are getting the right range of nutrients.

Folic acid

Adequate intake of folic acid is crucial for reducing the risk of birth defects associated with the brain and spinal cord. This nutrient, also known as folate, is a B vitamin (B9). In addition to eating a folate-rich diet, it is important to take folic acid supplements from the time you stop using contraception until the 12th week of pregnancy, when the risk of neural tube defects decreases. Recent studies have also confirmed a positive connection between folic acid and a reduction in the risk of childhood leukaemia.

The dose recommended for anyone who is pregnant or thinking of having a baby is 0.4mg (400mcg). As it is water soluble (and hence unable to be stored by your body) you may need a higher dose to ensure you have the right level of folate in your system. Consult your GP or midwife. For a list of foods containing folic acid, see the opposite page.

TAKING FOLIC ACID BEFORE YOU CONCEIVE

All babies are potentially at risk of developing spina bifida and other neural tube defects which affect the development of the brain and spinal cord. Defects mostly occur in the early stages of pregnancy, especially during the first 28 days when your baby's organs are developing, which is why it's vital to start taking folic acid before you discover you are pregnant. Folic acid plays a large role in cell growth and development as well as tissue formation. As you won't know at first if you are pregnant, it's important to begin taking folic acid supplements as soon as you start trying for a baby.

Feeling good – yes, it's possible!

ARE SOME WOMEN AT MORE RISK?

Women who've had twins or multiples or who have had babies close together may have a deficiency in certain vitamins and minerals, so it's important to start taking folic acid supplements well before falling pregnant again. Studies show that mothers who've had one child with a neural tube defect can decrease their risk of having another by 72% by taking folic acid supplements. If you have epilepsy, you may also require more folic acid and should consult your GP.

FOODS THAT CONTAIN FOLIC ACID INCLUDE:

- Broccoli
- Bananas
- Peas
- Kale
- Beans
- Cauliflower
- Baked beans
- Lentils
- Asparagus
- Citrus fruits
- Spinach
- Brussels sprouts
- Cabbage
- Potatoes
- Kiwi fruit
- Fortified breakfast cereals (check the labelling)
- Some breads (again, check the labelling)

If you are eating plenty of the above foods and taking the recommended daily dose of folic acid, you should be getting more than enough for your baby.

Protein

Protein is vital to sustain the rapid growth and development of your baby. Good sources of protein include: lean red meat, poultry, pulses, beans, soya beans, tofu, eggs and cheese. A word of caution about certain dairy products: pregnant women should avoid soft or 'mouldy' cheeses (such as Brie, Camembert and Stilton) due to the potential risk of listeria. In addition, make sure eggs are well cooked as there is always a slight risk of salmonella.

Carbohydrates

Carbohydrates are important in your diet, both to maintain your energy levels and to help your baby to grow. Try to cut back on refined carbohydrates such as white bread, rice and pasta, which have little nutritional benefit. Stock up instead on non-refined carbohydrates such as wholegrain cereals, wholegrain and rye bread, wholewheat pasta, and fruit and vegetables.

Calcium

Calcium – found in dairy produce, beans, chickpeas, tofu, tinned sardines and salmon (with bones), oats and certain greens – is crucial for the development of your baby's teeth and bones. It also helps to keep your muscles strong and healthy. If your body does not get enough of this mineral, your baby will use your calcium stores and then draw it from your bones.

Iron

Iron is needed to ensure a good supply of red blood cells, which transport oxygen to your baby and to your own muscles and organs. In pregnancy it is common to become anaemic (deficient in iron), especially if you are vegetarian, as vegetable sources of iron are more difficult for the body to process. Good sources of iron are to be found in lean red meat, wholegrain breads and cereals, beans, leafy green vegetables and dried fruits. Bear in mind, too, that vitamin C increases iron absorption, while tea (containing tannin) inhibits iron absorption and should be avoided if possible. Consult your GP if you think you may need iron supplements.

Selenium

Selenium is very important for vegetarians as it is an immune booster. While this trace mineral may be found in meat and fish, it also occurs in nuts, especially Brazil nuts, soya beans, cereals and eggs. Pregnant women in the UK will usually get all the selenium they need from their diet. Indeed, taken in excess – in doses higher than 400 mcg a day – selenium can be toxic. If, for whatever reason, you feel you need to take extra selenium, speak to your GP first.

Vitamin A

Vitamin A, important for maintaining good eyesight, is also essential for cell growth, tissue repair, bone formation and healthy skin, hair and teeth. However, it is not advisable to take vitamin A supplements as high doses may be harmful to your baby. Likewise, it is best to avoid eating liver (see page 50). If you are taking supplements, then beta-carotene (a nutrient that is converted to vitamin A by your body as required) is the best source. Most women receive all the vitamin A they need from their diet. The best food sources are carrots, dairy products, leafy green vegetables and sweet potatoes.

Vitamin B6

Vitamin B6, also known as pyridoxine, enables your body to obtain energy from the protein and carbohydrates that you eat. It is also helps oxygen-carrying haemoglobin to form. It will aid your baby's overall development and can help reduce morning sickness during the first trimester. The best food sources of B6 are salmon, eggs, green leafy vegetables, watermelons, bananas, soya beans, peanuts, milk, potatoes, bread, beef, pork and fortified breakfast cereals.

Vitamin B12

Vitamin B12 helps your body to process folic acid. It also assists in making red blood cells and keeping your nervous system healthy. This vitamin is found in poultry, red meat and fish, as well as in cheese, yeast and eggs. This may present a problem for a vegetarian, as there are limits to the amount of dairy foods you should be eating; hence it may be a good idea to take a supplement containing vitamin B12. If you're vegan, you may need supplementation too. Consult your GP or midwife for further advice.

Vitamin C

Vitamin C is essential for the development of your baby's skin, bones and tendons. It helps the body's tissues repair themselves and heightens your resistance to infection. It also helps your body to absorb iron properly. The best food sources of vitamin C are citrus fruits, kiwi fruit, broccoli, tomatoes, spinach and potatoes.

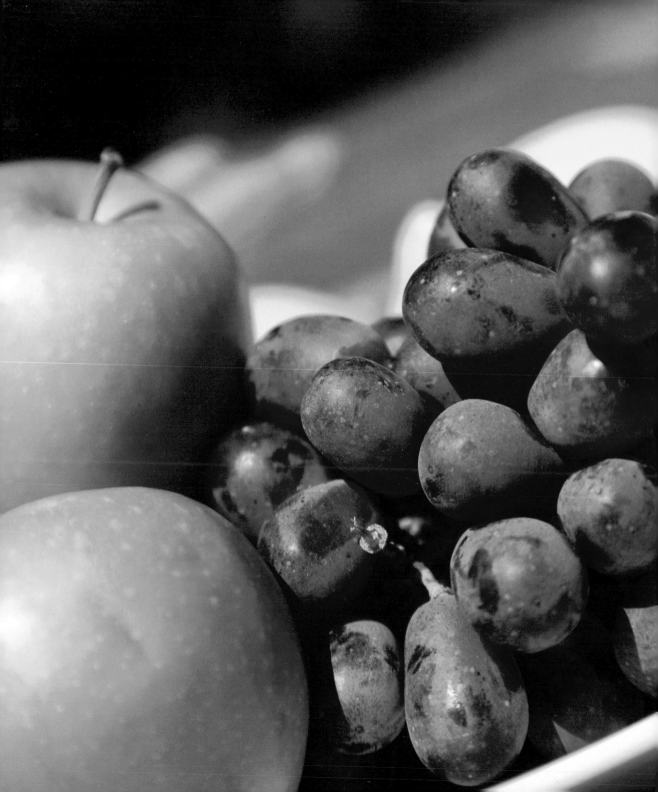

Vitamin D

Vitamin D is essential for effective calcium absorption. It is mostly obtained from sunlight as few foods contain it naturally, these being fish, liver and egg yolks. Fortified foods and drinks such as margarine and orange juice are otherwise the best dietary source. If you cover up your skin when you are outside (perhaps for religious reasons), it is wise to make sure you take around 10mcg per day as a supplement.

Antenatal supplements

If you have a good diet, you'll probably be getting enough nutrients and vitamins from what you eat. Specific pregnancy multivitamins are available if you think you need them (if you are vegetarian or suffer from bad morning sickness, for instance), but it's best to discuss with your doctor or midwife first and try to stick to a healthy, balanced diet.

Fluids

You are likely to feel thirstier than before you were pregnant and it's important to take in enough fluids so that you don't become dehydrated, making you feel tired, dizzy, hungry, and prone to headaches. Drink lots of water (preferably filtered or bottled) or go for herbal teas or fruit juices (preferably not from concentrate). Fluids to limit or avoid are caffeine-containing tea and coffee (try caffeine-free brands instead), and, of course, alcohol (see pages 48–53).

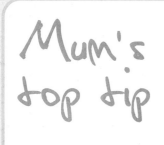

Mum's top tip

When I asked my midwife about any food supplements I should take, she suggested Omega 3 fish oils. These can be taken during pregnancy as long as they are free from retinol, the animal form of vitamin A. Alternatively, eating one or two portions of oily fish each week will give you the recommended intake of Omega 3 oils during pregnancy. Remember to avoid marlin, swordfish and shark due to the high levels of mercury they may contain.

Foods to avoid

While you are pregnant your immune system functions at a slightly lower level than normal, so you are at greater risk from infection and may need to watch what you eat. If you find that you have accidentally eaten the wrong thing, don't panic – the risks are small. Nonetheless, it is best to steer clear of certain foods for the time being.

CHEESE

Some cheese carries the risk of listeria, a bacterium that can cause serious problems for the mother and baby.

Avoid: Soft, mould-ripened cheeses such as Brie or Camembert, and blue-veined cheeses such as Danish Blue or Stilton. They can be eaten if they've been thoroughly cooked and are piping hot all the way through. Also avoid cheese made from unpasteurized sheep or goat's milk.

You can eat: Hard cheeses, such as Caerphilly, Cheddar, Cheshire, Derby, Double Gloucester, Edam, Emmental, Gouda, Gruyère, Halloumi, Parmesan and Pecorino (hard); soft and processed cheeses, including cottage cheese, cream cheese, mascarpone, mozzarella and processed cheese (such as cheese spread and slices).

FISH

Fish can contain high levels of the pollutant mercury, which can in turn affect the development of your baby's nervous system.

Avoid: Shark, swordfish and marlin. Limit your consumption of tuna to one fresh steak, or two cans, a week, and avoid raw fish such as sushi.

You can eat: Cod, plaice, haddock and oily fish such as mackerel.

SHELLFISH

Shellfish can contain bacteria that may cause food poisoning which can put you and your baby at risk.

Avoid: Raw or undercooked shellfish such as oysters, mussels, cold prawns and crab.

You can eat: Cooked shellfish.

MILK

Milk can carry the risk of listeria or toxoplasmosis.

Avoid: Green-top milk and unpasteurized sheep and goat's milk, unless it has been boiled for two minutes.

You can drink: Pasteurized, sterilized and UHT milk.

EGGS

Eggs can carry the risk of salmonella.

Avoid: Raw or runny eggs, mayonnaise made with raw egg (shop-bought mayonnaise is fine, but restaurants often make their own mayonnaise with raw egg, so always ask first) and mousses made with mayonnaise.

You can eat: Well-cooked eggs (so that the egg white and yolk are solid), commercially prepared mayonnaise and salad cream.

ICE CREAM

Ice cream can carry the risk of listeria.

Avoid: Homemade ice cream or soft-whipped ice cream from machines.

You can eat: Ice cream from cartons, but always check first that it does not contain raw eggs – some brands do.

MEAT AND POULTRY

Meat can carry a risk of toxoplasmosis, listeria and salmonella if it hasn't been cooked properly.

Avoid: Raw or undercooked meat (ask for your steaks to be well done for the next nine months and avoid Parma ham) and ready-cooked poultry unless it has been thoroughly reheated.
You can eat: Well-cooked meat and poultry.

LIVER

Liver can contain high levels of retinol (the animal form of vitamin A), which can be harmful to your developing baby.
Avoid: Liver or liver products such as liver sausage and pâté; fish oil supplements containing fish liver.

SALADS

Salads can carry the risk of listeria or toxoplasmosis if they haven't been washed properly. Some dressed salads, such as potato salad and coleslaw, may also contain raw egg.
Avoid: Packaged salads, unless you wash them first; ready-prepared, dressed salads such as coleslaw or potato salad.
You can eat: Any salad that has been properly washed.

COOKED-CHILLED FOODS

Cooked-chilled foods can carry the risk of listeria.
Avoid: Unheated cooked-chilled foods.
You can eat: Cooked-chilled foods that have been thoroughly heated all the way through.

PEANUTS

Peanuts can be dangerous if you or your partner's family has a history of peanut or other allergies, asthma, eczema or hayfever.
Avoid: Eating peanuts, or peanut products (satay chicken, for example) during pregnancy and while you are breastfeeding.
You can eat: Other nuts, such as walnuts or Brazil nuts.

CAFFEINE

Caffeine has been associated with a greater risk of miscarriage, and of your baby not growing properly. Government advice is to limit consumption to 300mg, about three cups a day.
Avoid: Drinking caffeine, or no more than 300mg a day. Bear in mind that energy drinks and chocolate also contain caffeine.

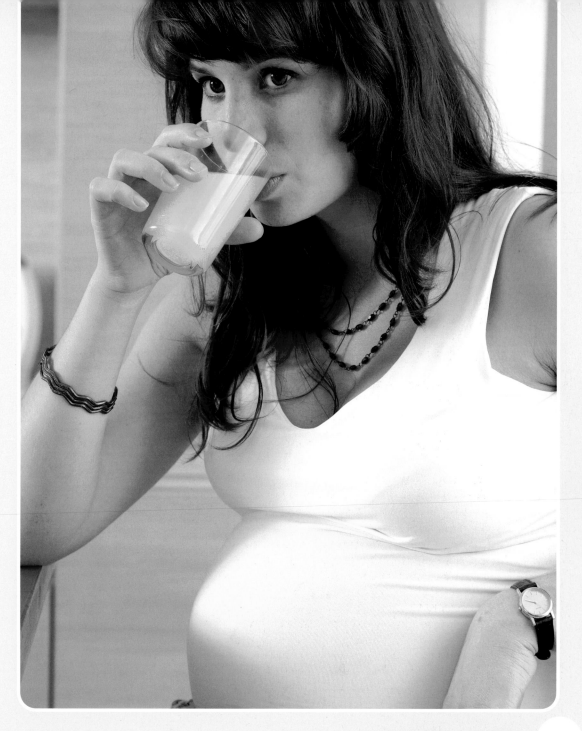

No drinking or smoking!

You may well find that you are at your most healthy during pregnancy because of the care and attention you pay to your lifestyle. There are a couple of definite no-nos for a healthy pregnancy, however. Follow this advice and you'll have nothing to regret.

Alcohol

Alcohol can be one of the hardest things to give up in early pregnancy, unless you find you can't stand the smell or taste of it, which makes giving up much easier! Recent government advice about alcohol consumption during pregnancy is that there is no safe level. This replaces previous advice that a couple of glasses of wine a week is not detrimental. The Department of Health issued these guidelines not on the basis of new research, but because of what it saw as a need to ensure pregnant women did not underestimate the potential risks to their baby.

HOW WILL MY BABY BE AFFECTED?

As alcohol passes through the placenta to the unborn child, potentially affecting his neurological development, women who continue to drink heavily throughout their pregnancies are putting their baby at serious risk. In extreme cases, the baby

Mum's top tip

Before I knew I was pregnant, I went on a girls' night out and had a couple of vodkas. As soon as I found out I was pregnant, the first thought I had was what effect the alcohol might have had on my baby. I felt so guilty and worried. My GP reassured me that there was unlikely to be a problem but I wanted to give my baby the best possible chance, so decided not to drink at all during my pregnancy.

may be born with foetal alcohol syndrome, a dangerous condition that inhibits growth, affects the nervous system and impairs learning and memory.

Smoking

Smoking is one of the most damaging things you can do to your unborn child, and the risks can be huge. It has been linked to miscarriage, stillbirth, low birthweight, damage to the placenta and a higher risk of foetal abnormalities. It is well documented that smoking during pregnancy increases the likelihood of pregnancy complications as well.

If your partner smokes, he is compromising the baby's health through your passive smoking. In addition, as smoking can lower a man's sperm count, it is advisable that he stops smoking even before you try for a baby.

If you smoke during pregnancy, you are putting your baby at risk of:
- Being born premature
- Having a low birthweight
- Cot death (also known as sudden infant death syndrome)
- Childhood cancers
- Meningococcal infections
- Middle ear infections
- Mental and intellectual deficiencies
- Respiratory problems such as asthma
- Childhood hyperactivity

The reason that smoking is so bad for your baby is that he is effectively being poisoned by carbon monoxide each time you light up. This means that less oxygen can reach him, with potentially highly damaging effects. He has no choice about this, whereas you have a choice not to impose this on him. If you manage to quit before the fourth month of pregancy, the risk to your baby is hugely reduced; even giving up later in pregnancy can help reduce the ill effects on your baby. It is never too late to give up!

Cravings during pregnancy

Most women find that during pregnancy they crave certain foods. It's believed that these cravings may be associated with their dietary needs at this time.

For example, a desire for chocolate or other sweet things may reflect your need for more calories during pregnancy – although it is fairly obvious that indulging in such foods is not the most nutritious way to obtain more calories!

Common cravings include fruit, pickles (onions, gherkins, etc.), crisps, and milk or dairy products. Reports of strange cravings during pregnancy, especially odd combinations such as pickles with ice cream, are rife. However, if you are experiencing slightly more unusual cravings – especially for non-food items such as coal, plaster or soap – this may be a sign that you are lacking important minerals or nutrients in your diet, in particular iron, and it is advisable to consult your GP or midwife. They should be able to test for any deficiencies and offer supplementation if necessary.

Thanks to all those hormones unleashed in your system during pregnancy, your appetite at this time may change dramatically. Your sense of smell and of taste may be heightened; you may experience extreme hunger pangs one day and an aversion to any number of different foods or drinks the next. One of the signs of pregnancy is a sudden inability to tolerate a particular food (especially one with a strong smell) that you enjoyed eating pre-pregnancy.

This is all perfectly normal, and it is only really when your appetite impacts on your nutritional intake that you need to worry. If you are famished and gorge on unhealthy 'quick fix' energy foods such as cakes, biscuits and crisps, then you need to have a rethink about your diet. Likewise, if your appetite is affected to the point where you cannot bring yourself to eat, you may be depriving your baby of important nutrients and should therefore speak to your GP about it.

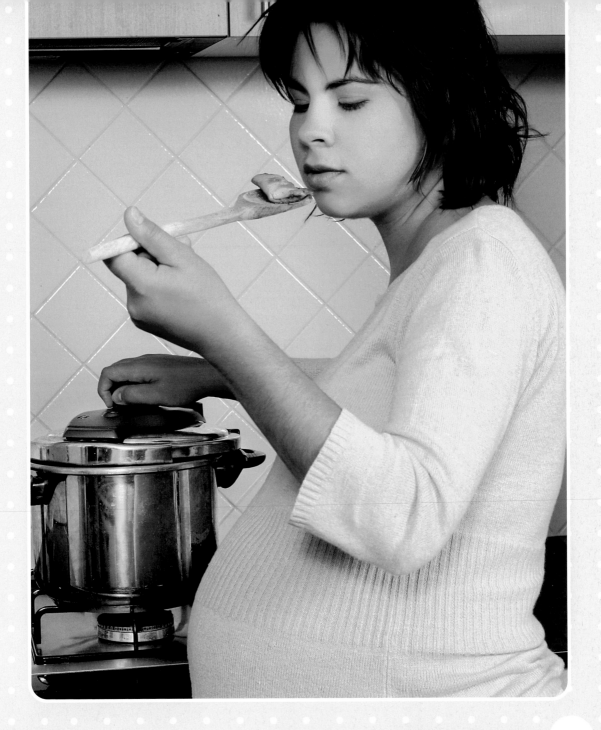

Exercise during pregnancy

Thankfully, pregnancy is no longer viewed as an illness and women have, in the main, stopped being treated as invalids. Nowadays, so long as your pregnancy is proceeding well, moderate physical exercise is seen as beneficial. Before you start, however, it is essential that you receive approval from your doctor. If you are in a high-risk category of pregnancy, you may have to avoid exercise. If not, then any exercise you take up should be low impact, just to be on the safe side.

If you are already physically fit and used to exercising, it is likely that you will be able to continue your routine, perhaps modifying it slightly. If you are new to serious exercise, pregnancy may not be the time to start. It is important to consult your GP before embarking on an exercise programme.

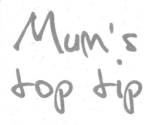

I found that exercise was a great way to combat mood swings and boost my flagging energy levels. I began an antenatal yoga class, which you can start after you have reached 12 weeks of pregnancy. Pregnancy yoga is a great way to meet other mums and to get to know your changing body and feel good about it. I also found that lots of fresh air helped me sleep better, so would take a short stroll round the block every day.

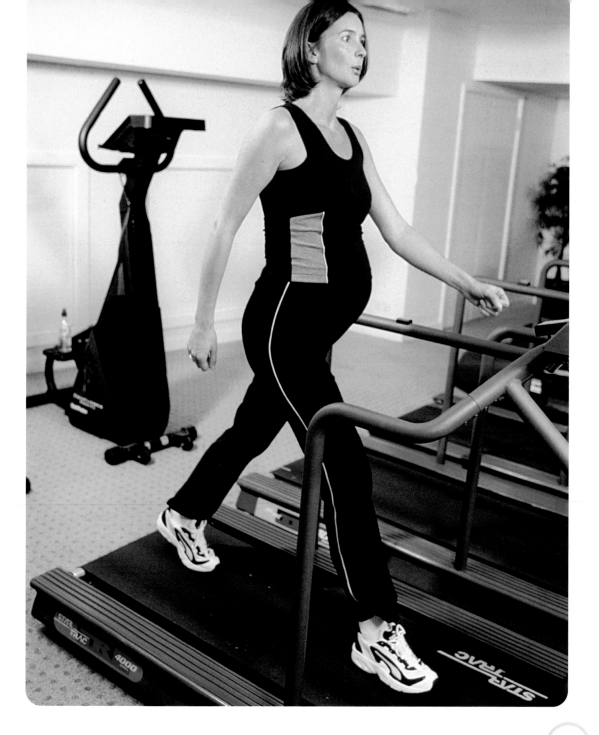

You should warm up with gentle stretches for ten minutes before attempting any serious exercise. In the beginning, the main activity should be limited to only five minutes, which you can then increase as your fitness grows. It's important not to get hot, out of breath or sweaty now that you are pregnant, as the increase in your body temperature could be bad for your baby. If at any time you experience ANY discomfort, then STOP exercising immediately and consult your GP before resuming your routine.

Swimming

As a safe and gentle way to exercise your body during pregnancy, swimming is ideal. The water supports your body and you can move at your own pace. Choose between swimming lengths or joining an antenatal water class. Held at many public pools, these special classes offer a chance to meet other mums-to-be as well as enjoy a gentle exercise routine.

Cycling

A great form of aerobic exercise – along with swimming and brisk walking – cycling stimulates the heart and lungs and helps to build muscle tone. It also increases your ability to process and utilize oxygen, a definite bonus for your baby. The safest way to do this is on a stationary bicycle (an exercise bike), so the risk of falling is reduced. Extreme caution should be taken on a normal bike; not only could bad weather conditions make a fall more likely but there is a greater risk of accidents. In the later stages of pregnancy, it is advisable to avoid any type of cycling as the weight of your baby may affect your balance.

Walking

This is one of the easiest and cheapest ways to keep fit. Brisk walking for half an hour a day is a good alternative to joining an exercise class or going to the pool. Why not vary your routine by visiting a local park or going for a walk in the country with a friend?

Yoga

Yoga is one of the most popular choices of exercise for pregnant women. Not only does it help to relax and unwind the body and mind, but the gentle stretches and focus on breathing are key components in preparing the body for labour.

Some people believe that this type of physical training helps women to actively take control over their labour, reducing the need for pain relief by helping them relax and accept the process rather than being fearful and tensing up. During antenatal yoga classes, muscles are also strengthened and there is often an emphasis on firming up the pelvic floor, reducing the likelihood of stitches and therefore speeding postpartum recovery.

Many places, including community centres and leisure centres, offer yoga classes for pregnant women. Ask your midwife for details of the nearest classes in your area.

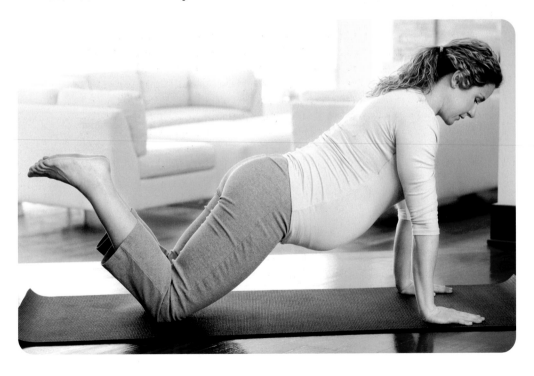

Exercise: how much is too much?

Olympic athlete Paula Radcliffe may have run right up until the day she went into hospital to have her first child, daughter Isla, but for the rest of us mere mortals such strenuous exercise during pregnancy is not generally recommended.

In the first five months of her pregnancy, Paula reportedly continued training at a level most athletes who aren't pregnant would find daunting, running for 75 minutes every morning and 30-45 minutes every evening, including hill work. But she was closely monitored by her doctor throughout and given an ultrasound once a month to ensure her pregnancy was progressing normally.

Maintaining a certain level of fitness during pregnancy is important but you must be careful not to overdo it. Regular exercise during pregnancy will help you stay relaxed and calm and tone your leg muscles, which means you'll find certain labour positions, such as squatting, less taxing. And the fitter you are before birth, the easier you will find the birth, as well as regaining your pre-birth body.

The type of exercise usually recommended during pregnancy, however, is of the gentle variety, such as swimming, yoga and walking. But what if you're used to doing more, and gentle workouts just aren't enough for you? There are medical concerns that strenuous exercise can increase the likelihood of miscarriage. Clearly, it is advisable to avoid any form of exercise where there is a chance that you could injure yourself, so skiing, horse-riding, roller-blading, ice-skating, trampolining and climbing are all out. Strenuous types of exercise such as high-impact aerobics, and contact sports like football, rugby, netball or lacrosse are also best avoided for obvious reasons. The same goes for extreme sports such as scuba-diving and parachuting.

However, there is light at the end of the tunnel if you have your heart set on continuing an exercise regime which doesn't consist solely of lots of deep breaths, 'ohms' and gentle strolls in the park. If you were very fit before pregnancy then it is possible you will be able to continue with the sport you're passionate about. For instance, if you are an avid runner you should be able to continue jogging. What's crucial, however, is that you consult your GP first. You may be advised to adopt a modified version of your favourite exercise during your first trimester. Then, as you enter your second trimester, you will probably be advised to take it down another notch.

Even if your doctor has given you the all-clear to continue exercising during pregnancy, it's important that you stop immediately if you experience any of the following symptoms:
- Palpitations
- Dizziness
- Exhaustion
- Breathlessness
- Aches and pains
- Vaginal bleeding.

Morning sickness

Approximately half of all pregnant women will experience some type of sickness during their pregnancy. This is believed to be due to the high levels of the pregnancy hormone, HCG, in your system. Most often, the 'sickness' refers to feeling nauseous but it can involve episodes of vomiting. Fortunately, it is usually more of a problem in the first trimester (the first three months), after which your hormone levels settle down and any sickness usually goes away.

'Morning' sickness can be misleading: for some women the nausea is thankfully confined to the early hours, however for those who are less fortunate the sickness can continue throughout the day. Sickness usually subsides after the first three months, although for an unlucky few, it continues throughout all three trimesters.

Top tips to help you cope with morning sickness

1 Try to drink plenty of fluids, especially if you are vomiting a lot. It's important not to get dehydrated as this can be harmful for both you and your baby. Take small sips of water rather than gulping and, if you think you can handle it, try drinking a few sips of a sports energy drink to replace lost sugars.

2 Avoid the aroma and sight of foods that make your stomach turn. If the smell of frying bacon sends you hurtling towards the bathroom, simply ban it from the house. Talk to your partner, family or housemates and explain the situation – you will be surprised at how understanding they can be.

top
tips

Feeling good – yes, it's possible!

3 Eating a dry biscuit or piece of toast on waking, before lying down for half an hour, can help to alleviate the symptoms of sickness. Ginger is recognized as a sickness combatant, so stock up on ginger biscuits and keep them in your bedside table or drawer at work so you can have a nibble when you feel hungry, as feeling hungry often makes the nausea worse.

4 Foods high in starch, such as bread and potatoes, may help to keep up blood sugar levels and make you feel full. If you can, stick to bland foods rather than fatty, acidic or spicy ones that are harder to digest and may irritate your digestive system.

5 This is the time to forget about dieting. If you suffer badly from sickness and all you feel like eating is chips – just do it. Morning sickness is temporary, after all. If you don't manage to get food into you, of any kind, serious problems can occur and you may end up in hospital. As long as you are not eating any foods considered unsafe in pregnancy (see pages 48–51), this is a time when anything goes.

6 If you are travelling on public transport, allow extra time to get to work in case you have to leave the train/bus to get some air before catching the next one. Take ginger biscuits to nibble on throughout your journey and keep yourself occupied with a magazine, book or some music.

Mum's top tip

When I had morning sickness with my last pregnancy, I felt queasy the whole time and the smell of food made me feel worse. I found that if I ate something *before* I felt really sick, it helped the nausea stay away. The trick for me was not to get too hungry. I found things like plain biscuits, toast or cream crackers with a little butter and a drink of lemonade really settled my morning sickness and made it much more bearable.

top tips

Mood swings

Pregnancy forces huge changes onto you, both physical and psychological. Suddenly you have to deal with the responsibility of a new life growing inside you. You're likely to worry about whether you are eating or doing the right things and about the impact the baby will have on your life, your work and your relationships. With the added effects of pregnancy hormones flowing around your body, it's hardly surprising that your moods are constantly fluctuating.

Antenatal depression

Mood swings are perfectly normal and usually settle down when you reach the second trimester. If you are feeling constantly anxious or depressed, however, you may be experiencing antenatal depression, which affects roughly 10% of women. A study carried out by the *British Medical Journal* has suggested that antenatal depression may be even more common than postnatal depression (following the birth of the baby) and should be taken just as seriously. Your doctor or midwife can help you with this if you are concerned. It is worth remembering that the symptoms of antenatal depression are different from the normal mood swings experienced during pregnancy. Antenatal depression is much more acute, affecting your day-to-day life. You might need medication (your doctor will make sure it's safe for you to take) to help you feel better. Seek help sooner rather than later, and remember that your doctor (or midwife) will have encountered it many times before.

TYPICAL SYMPTOMS INCLUDE:

- Anxiety
- Extreme irritability with others as well as yourself
- Inability to concentrate on anything
- Extreme tiredness (bearing in mind that extreme tiredness is in itself a symptom of early pregnancy)
- Inability to sleep
- Inability to eat and lack of appetite
- Inability to enjoy anything or feeling constantly sad or upset
- Not wanting to leave the house or socialize with anyone
- Obsessive-compulsive tendencies – repeating actions such as washing your hands or turning lights on and off

Accept your feelings and share them

The first thing to do is to acknowledge that you are not superwoman. We all have expectations about how we would like to experience pregnancy and sometimes we are too hard on ourselves. Images of young, beautiful celebrities sailing through pregnancy with effortless grace have become a familiar sight in recent times. However, these images are only that: images. You would not be human if you did not feel a whole range of different emotions at different points during your pregnancy. You are not a robot and you haven't been airbrushed! Accept that this is a time of great change, both mentally and physically, and you will realize that this conflict of emotions is actually perfectly normal.

Explain to your partner how you are feeling rather than bottling it all up and then taking it out on him. Although you might feel that you are going through pregnancy on your own, it is definitely worth sharing how you feel with your partner. The chances are he'll be sharing some of the same anxieties and it will help if you explain to him that you've been feeling low. Also, talk to your GP or midwife, or someone else you can trust, about how you are feeling.

Sex during pregnancy

Sex can be a source of anxiety during pregnancy as many couples worry that it will be harmful to their developing baby. You may be concerned that intercourse or having an orgasm will hurt your baby or bring on early labour, but unless you have been advised not to have sex by your GP or midwife, there is no reason why you shouldn't enjoy a healthy sex life. While you are pregnant your uterus is sealed by a mucus plug that protects your baby from infection.

During pregnancy there is an increased blood flow around your pelvic area due to hormonal changes. This can induce a heightened sense of arousal and give rise to longer orgasms. You may also feel greater sensitivity in your nipples and breasts. Indeed, rather than sex being harmful to your baby, some research suggests that babies actually benefit from their parents making love because of the increase in oxygen generated in the womb.

Mum's top tip

It's natural to go off sex in the first trimester, especially if you are feeling tired and sick. But I found that when I got to about 15 weeks my sex drive returned, even more powerfully than before! All fours can be a good position in the later stages of pregnancy when your bump is getting big. You kneel on all fours and your partner kneels behind you. Make sure your arms, not your stomach, are taking your weight.

Tender breasts can make sex uncomfortable, but this is not usually a problem until later in pregnancy. Colostrum, the first milk you produce, can leak from your breasts when you are aroused (or when you hear a baby crying) but, again, this is not usually a problem until the later stages of pregnancy.

Because of the hormonal changes in your body, the consistency, volume and odour of your vaginal discharge will probably change during pregnancy. This can mean an increase in lubrication which in turn can be beneficial for lovemaking.

Oral sex is perfectly safe during pregnancy, as long as your partner is careful not to blow into your vagina. This could force air into your bloodstream and be dangerous for you and your baby.

When should sex be avoided in pregnancy?

- If you have a tendency to miscarry, it may be wise to abstain from sex until you are past 12 weeks.

- If you have a history of pre-term labour, or are experiencing signs of early labour, it may be suggested that you avoid sex in the last trimester.

- If you have placenta praevia (a low-lying placenta), avoid sex in the last trimester.

- If you experience any vaginal bleeding, stop having sex and see your doctor or midwife as soon as possible.

Maternity clothes

Before your bump appears you'll probably be inspecting your tummy every morning to work out whether there's any sign of it yet. Don't worry, you'll see it soon!

When your bump starts to show depends entirely on you and your body shape. If you are tall your bump may not appear until around the five-month mark; by contrast, if you are small it may appear after only a month. Everyone is different, so you'll just have to wait and see. By month six, most women will be throwing down their skinny jeans in horror and shopping for something looser and more comfortable.

It's not just your belly that changes during pregnancy, it's your legs, breasts, feet, arms, bum and hips too! Thankfully most women go back to something near their old shape over the first year of their baby's life, although the majority do report that their figures have changed from pre-pregnancy – often for the better!

So, how to go about buying maternity clothes? Thankfully most clothing stores have stylish and affordable maternity ranges and plenty of styles to suit all budgets. The trick is to select key pieces to last you through pregnancy. (For more on high-street retailers selling maternity clothing, see Resources, pages 216–17.)

Maternity-wear hints and tips

top tips

1 Buy your own size
When buying maternity clothes, don't be tempted to buy ones that are too big; stick to the size you were before pregnancy. This is because maternity clothes will allow for the bump while hopefully fitting you perfectly everywhere else.

2 Keep it simple and comfortable
When investing in new maternity clothes, try to keep it simple. Buy two pairs of trousers, three tops and two vests to start with.

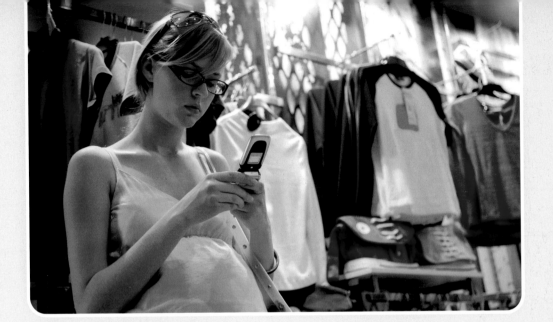

You can always buy more if you feel you need them further along the line. Invest in some funky new accessories too – they can completely change the look of an outfit. If you are trying a maternity outfit on and it's a little tight or restrictive – don't buy it! You're only going to get bigger and you need to allow room for growth. It's best to put comfort first during this time.

3 Invest in a good bra and knickers

Well-fitting, comfortable maternity bras and knickers are essential. Some women can get away with wearing their normal knickers as their bump fits over the top; others may find their pre-pregnancy styles restrictive. Maternity knickers, especially those with a high percentage of cotton, are the most comfortable option. In addition, it's crucial to wear the right kind of bra during pregnancy because your breasts will almost certainly get bigger, necessitating more support. Don't buy an underwired bra because the wires can interfere with the delicate milk ducts that are in the process of forming. If you plan to breastfeed, it's probably best to wait until after your baby is born and your milk has come in before you buy a nursing bra as your breasts will get bigger still!

top tips

Getting the best antenatal care

What is antenatal care?

Antenatal check-ups are very much something to look forward to. Not only do they provide an opportunity to have your questions answered and your fears allayed, they keep you up to date on your health and your baby's physical progress as well.

The number of appointments you have with your midwife will vary depending on whether this is your first pregnancy, whether you have any complications and what type of midwife care you have opted for (see overleaf).

There are official recommendations as to how many antenatal checks you should receive. According to guidelines from the NHS's National Institute of Clinical Excellence (NICE), a woman who has never given birth before may expect a schedule of ten antenatal appointments, while a woman who has previously experienced an uncomplicated birth will typically be offered a schedule of seven.

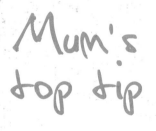

When I was first pregnant, I must admit that I found all the different antenatal care options rather confusing. The best thing to do when you're first pregnant, I think, is to chat to other mums who live near to you about the different antenatal care on offer in your area and, from there, decide which of the options suits you best. It really helped me!

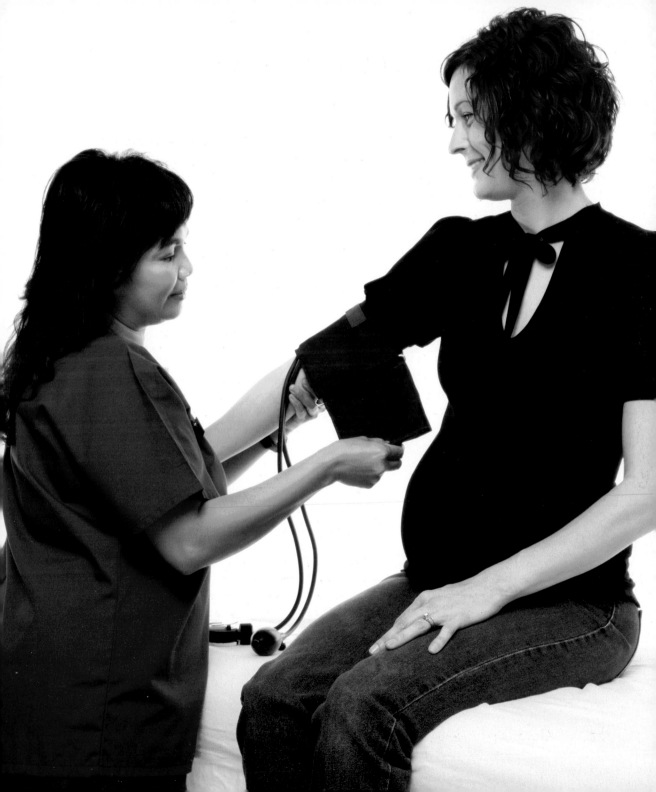

Antenatal care: who provides it?

YOUR GP
Usually the first professional carer that you will encounter after discovering you are pregnant is your GP. Your doctor is responsible for confirming your pregnancy and referring you to the relevant healthcare professionals and local hospital.

YOUR OBSTETRICIAN
The job of an obstetrician is to deal with any medical complications or problems that may arise during pregnancy or delivery. With luck, you will never need to see your obstetrician although you will be assigned one who is attached to the hospital you have been referred to and where you will give birth (unless you opt for a home delivery, see pages 118–21).

YOUR CONSULTANT
If you are experiencing a pregnancy with complications, or you had complications in a previous pregnancy, you may have to see a consultant for your antenatal checks. Most women who have uncomplicated pregnancies see a midwife and their GP.

YOUR MIDWIVES
Unless there is a particular midwife attached to your antenatal clinic who you see at each visit, or unless you have an independent midwife, it is likely that you will see different midwives throughout your pregnancy. They will help you to make informed choices about your care before and during the birth, carry out clinical examinations and provide you with important information to help you through pregnancy.

Midwives work in the maternity section of general hospitals, in private maternity hospitals and in group practices, at birth centres and with GPs. They look after women in many different circumstances and from all different walks of life.

If you feel it is important to have continuous care from one person throughout your pregnancy, it might be worth investigating the cost and practicality of employing an independent midwife.

An independent midwife is a registered midwife who is self-employed on either a full- or part-time basis. She provides care for you in the place that you choose: at your home or local hospital. For women who would prefer not to be seen by a different midwife each time, an independent midwife may be the answer.

Your midwife will be one of the most important people you see during your pregnancy, at your labour and for a short period postnatally. She (or he) will usually be your first port of call for information as your pregnancy develops, and she will be able to advise you on all aspects of pregnancy, labour, birth and looking after your baby.

Independent midwives will normally be present during your antenatal care and also at the birth. If you are interested in investigating this type of caregiver further, contact the Independent Midwives Association (see Resources, pages 216–17, for contact details).

What happens at antenatal check-ups?

BLOOD PRESSURE

At each antenatal appointment, your blood pressure will be taken to check for conditions such as pre-eclampsia (see pages 102-3). Your blood pressure should be slightly lower than before or after pregnancy; it should not be above 140/90. If it is high, it can be controlled by blood pressure tablets, and regular antenatal checks will be advised.

URINE

Most clinics will require you to give a urine sample at every antenatal visit. Your urine is tested for a number of things. Most importantly, your sugar levels are checked for gestational diabetes (see pages 98-99), your protein levels for hyper-tension, and ketone levels to see how your kidneys are coping.

BLOOD TESTS

Blood tests will be carried out at various points during your pregnancy. Typically they will happen at your first visit, at around 15 weeks, at 24-26 weeks (during your glucose test) and at 34 weeks. Blood tests provide screening for conditions such as HIV, syphilis, hepatitis B, sickle-cell anaemia and iron-deficiency anaemia. The early blood test at around 15 weeks is designed to screen for conditions such as Down's syndrome (see pages 93-5) and spina bifida.

PHYSICAL EXAMINATION

Depending on your antenatal clinic, you may or may not have a physical examination at the start of your pregnancy. More than likely, you will be weighed and your height will be measured. During your first visit, you will be asked about your family medical history and your general health.

INTERNAL EXAMINATION

You will probably not need an internal examination unless it is deemed necessary.

YOUR BABY'S HEARTBEAT

From about week 14, it should be possible to hear your baby's heartbeat. The midwife will listen to it with a foetal Doppler – a special hand-held device which measures your baby's heartbeat through your abdomen. If your baby is a wriggler, it can be hard to locate the heartbeat, but don't worry; even if it takes time, your midwife will find it!

PALPATION

Palpation is the act of feeling your abdomen, by your GP or midwife, to discover how your baby is lying in the womb, the size of your belly and also if he has engaged (moved head-down into the pelvic cavity) in the last stages of pregnancy.

Other tests and checks

In addition to the tests conducted routinely at antenatal appointments, a range of other checks and tests are available. These fall into different categories, including blood screening tests, diagnostic tests and ultrasound scans (see pages 84–9). Most women are offered at least one ultrasound scan during pregnancy, at about 20 weeks. Sometimes an earlier scan is conducted, taking place at around 12 weeks. These scans help detect any problems and give you a picture of your growing baby.

Mum's top tip

I found my midwife was one of the most important people I saw during my first pregnancy and when she visited me at home with my baby. She was my first port of call for information as my pregnancy developed, and she was able to advise me on all aspects of pregnancy and looking after my baby. I kept a notebook to jot down any questions that occurred to me between appointments – my memory became a sieve during pregnancy!

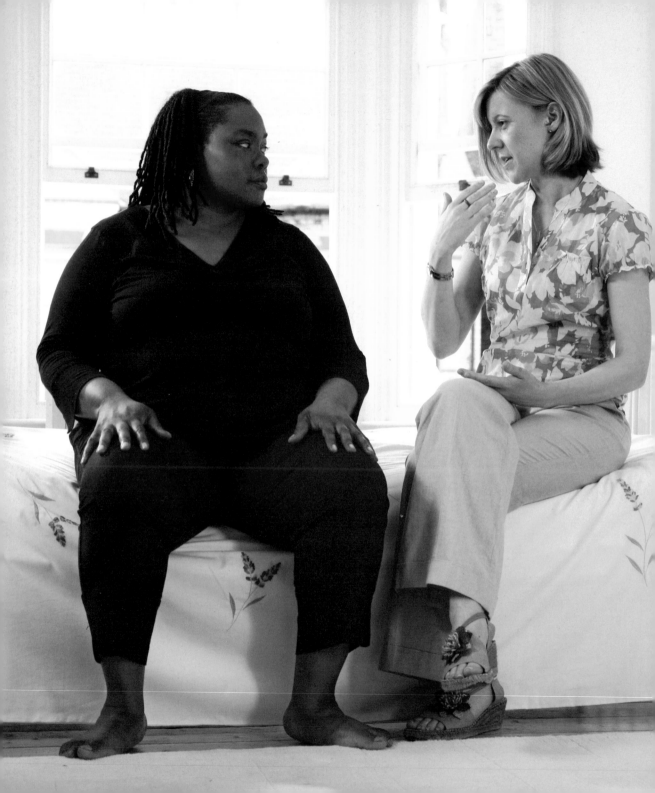

Shared care

Many women opt for shared care, which is when you visit both your midwife and your GP for antenatal appointments. It can be beneficial in the later stages of pregnancy to be able to go to your GP if the surgery is close to home.

When you see your midwife or GP, you should always tell them about any concerns you may have, from swelling ankles or varicose veins to piles or just feeling uncomfortable.

Birth doulas

'Doula' is a Greek word meaning 'female servant' or 'caregiver'. A doula is not necessarily a trained midwife but should have a good physiological understanding of pregnancy and ideally a lot of experience of childbirth. A doula does not offer clinical support in the way that a midwife, GP or obstetrician does; the emphasis is much more on emotional support. For this reason, women sometimes choose their friends or mothers to be their birth doula.

The job of the doula is to offer emotional and practical support throughout the birth and afterwards. This might include preparatory antenatal meetings and sometimes meeting up postnatally too. Recent research in the US has suggested that the number of Caesarean births could be halved, time spent in labour could be cut by 25% and forceps delivery reduced by 40% if women had the support of a doula during labour and birth.

During the birth, the doula will offer comfort and reassurance to the mother and may also involve the father in the process. The belief is that a woman can be empowered through her experience of childbirth, regarding it in a much more positive light, if she receives this kind of support. The presence of the doula is believed to lessen pain, shorten first-time labour, decrease the need for surgical intervention and increase the success rate of breastfeeding. If you are interested in finding out more information about birth doulas, contact Doula UK (see Resources, pages 216–17, for details).

Maternity notes understood

The strange list of abbreviations that appear on your maternity notes can be quite baffling, so here is a guide to what some of them mean:

Alb: Albumin in urine

AFP: Alpha-fetoprotein

BP: Blood pressure

Br: Breech (your baby is lying with his legs down)

Ceph: Cephalic (your baby is lying head down)

CS: Caesarean section

EDD/EDC: Estimated date of delivery/confinement

Eng/E: Engaged (your baby's head is sitting in the pelvis)

Fe: Iron prescribed

FH: Foetal heart

FHH/NH: Foetal heart heard or not heard

FMF: Foetal movements felt

Hb: Haemoglobin levels to check for anaemia

Height of fundus: The height of the top of the uterus

H/T: Hypertension (high blood pressure)

Long L: Longitudinal lie (your baby lies parallel to your spine in the uterus)

LMP: Last menstrual period

MSU: Midstream urine sample

Multigravida: You have had more than one pregnancy

NAD: No abnormality detected

NE: Not engaged

Oed: Oedema

PET: Pre-eclamptic toxaemia

Primigravida: This is your first pregnancy

Relation of PP to brim: This refers to the brim of your pelvis. The PP is the presenting part of the baby, which will be born first

RSA: Right sacrum anterior. This is the most common breech presentation

TCA: To come again

VE: Vaginal examination

Getting the best antenatal care

Concerns during pregnancy

If you have any concerns between appointments, it's usually possible to get in touch with your midwife to ask for her advice. Ask your midwife at your first appointment about how to contact her as different areas operate different systems. If you are having problems getting in touch with your midwife or making an earlier appointment, you should make an appointment with your GP as soon as possible. Do not suffer in silence, as you may find yourself becoming stressed and worrying needlessly about things. Seek advice and have your mind put at rest as soon as you can.

Remember that it's common to have concerns when you're pregnant, especially if it's your first pregnancy. Here we've provided a list of the top concerns of an expectant mum, to reassure you that you're not alone in your worries!

1 Am I providing my baby with the correct nutrients?
It's important to consume a healthy, well-balanced diet during pregnancy (see pages 42–7 for more details).

2 Are these twinges normal?
Many women experience twinges during pregnancy. If these are intense in nature or accompanied by bleeding or severe abdominal cramping, you should consult a doctor immediately.

3 Could the antibiotics I took or alcohol I consumed before I found out I was pregnant have harmed my unborn baby?
Many women worry about this, but the likelihood is that your baby will be fine. The important thing is to give up, or cut down to a minimum, your consumption of alcohol and caffeine once you realize you're pregnant. It's also advised that you give up smoking completely. (For more information on what to avoid in pregnancy, see pages 48–51 and 52–3.)

4 Can I still exercise in pregnancy?

As well as being concerned about what they eat, women worry about what forms of exercise are safe in pregnancy. Gentle exercise is extremely beneficial (see pages 56–9).

5 Which childhood infections could harm my unborn baby?

As long as you're vigilant, you shouldn't have cause to worry, but you should try to avoid coming into contact with children who have chicken pox or rubella (German measles).

6 Will I be sufficiently prepared for labour?

It's normal to feel somewhat apprehensive about labour. It's therefore important to do your research and, if you can, attend antenatal classes (see page 110) so you feel as prepared as possible. Do ask your midwife or GP if you are feeling concerned about labour and birth or if you have any questions about how the birth will be managed.

7 Will the changes to my body be permanent?

Your body's likely to change dramatically during pregnancy but, for the most part, everything will return to how it was before you were pregnant. If you are worried about stretch marks, you may want to massage your tummy with oil to minimize them.

8 How will I know if I am in labour?

This is a question that many women worry about. It's is best to ask your midwife so that you know exactly what to expect (see page 160).

9 Will I be able to breastfeed?

Many women believe that for one reason or another they won't be able to breastfeed, but most women can. Ask your midwife about any concerns you have and where you can get information about and help with breastfeeding.

10 Will I be able to tell if my baby's ill?

Your newborn baby will be more prone to infection as his immune system won't have fully matured. Look out for any changes in his behaviour – whether he's crying more than usual, for instance – and contact your GP if you are at all worried.

Ten questions to ask your midwife

1 What can I do to ensure my baby and I stay healthy during pregnancy?

2 Based on my health and family medical history, what complications could occur in my pregnancy?

3 When will my antenatal checks be?

4 What tests will I have and when will I have my first scan?

5 Is it safe to drink alcohol during pregnancy?

6 What are my birthing options based on my pregnancy so far?

7 When can I book antenatal or childbirth preparation classes?

8 Can I get in contact with you if I have concerns between appointments?

9 Who can be present at the birth of my baby?

10 What pain relief methods are most women offered?

Mum's top tip

My advice is to keep your maternity notes with you at all times so that if you see a different caregiver, then he or she has all the information to hand. He will read about what happened at your last antenatal appointment, check your blood pressure and any medication you are taking. If you have any concerns, mention them to him so that he can decide what treatment, if any, is needed.

Antenatal scans

A range of scans may be performed during pregnancy, some routine, some not. This section looks at the different types of scan that you may be offered.

Ultrasound scans

An ultrasound scan sends sound waves through the body, which are then reflected back and converted into an image that is visible on a screen. In the UK this is a routine procedure during pregnancy. Most parents-to-be relish being able to see their baby for the first time in this way, especially the father, who may have a more abstract notion of the pregnancy. It is an opportunity to make the experience of becoming a parent more of a reality.

Scans can reveal the sex of your baby, although they are not always 100% accurate and so should not be wholly relied upon for this purpose. There are countless stories of parents who were informed during a scan that their baby was a boy, only to get a shock when 'he' was born a she! Similarly, little problems are sometimes missed and occasionally major issues go unnoticed. The effectiveness of the scan will depend on the quality of the equipment, the diagnostic ability of the sonographer and the position in which your baby is lying in the womb. The key thing to remember is that an ultrasound scan is a screening and not a diagnostic device. If anything shows up during the scan that the sonographer is concerned about, you will be referred for further tests. An ultrasound scan can provide a good overall idea of how your baby is developing, but even the finest examination cannot detect every possible problem.

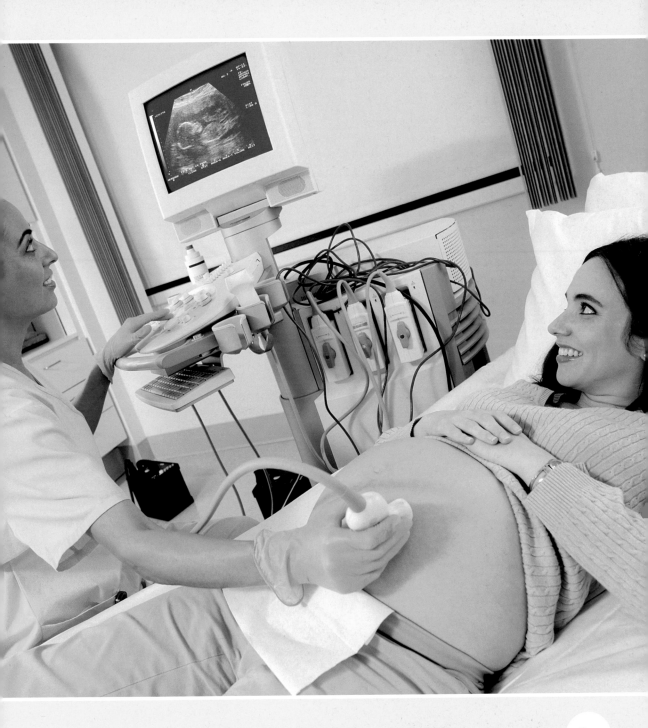

WHAT HAPPENS AT AN ULTRASOUND SCAN?

If you are having a scan, you need to drink plenty of water beforehand. If your bladder is full, this enables the sonographer to get a much better picture of your uterus. You lie on your back and the sonographer puts some clear gel on your stomach to help the transducer probe move easily over your skin. If you are having a scan in early pregnancy (around 12 weeks), it may not be possible to pick up much because your baby is still too small. If this is the case, you may be offered a vaginal scan. Known as transvaginal ultrasonography, this is a painless procedure in which a small probe is placed inside your vagina to obtain a clearer picture of how your baby is growing.

The sonographer should talk you through what he or she is doing and you can ask questions about what you can see on the screen. Usually, you are able to keep the picture of the scan; sometimes you may be asked to donate a small fee for it.

An early scan will check your baby's heartbeat and that she is developing normally. The sonographer will be able to see your baby's head, arms and legs and some internal organs. Checking for any abnormalities and growth problems cannot be carried out at this stage but must wait until your 20-week scan.

CAN THE ULTRASOUND DETECT WHAT SEX MY BABY IS?

By about 18–20 weeks, an ultrasound can identify the sex of your baby, if you want to know. If you don't want to know, it might be a good idea to tell the sonographer straight away in case you accidentally get a glimpse!

Babies frequently won't oblige, in any case. If your baby is turning away from the sonographer and you can't get a clear enough picture of the genitals, you may have to wait until the birth to find out. Even the best sonographers can't guarantee 100% that your baby is a boy or a girl, so don't go too mad decorating the nursery a particular colour or buying baby clothes until you have your baby in your arms.

Dating scan

If you are unsure about your dates and are unable to establish when you fell pregnant, it is likely that you will be offered an ultrasound scan to find out your conception date.

Scans carried out during the first 13 weeks of pregnancy are incredibly accurate at establishing this information. If, for whatever reason, you are opposed to having an ultrasound scan, you may be offered an internal examination, which can also ascertain how many weeks pregnant you are.

WHEN WILL I HAVE A DATING SCAN?

Women tend to be offered a dating scan at around 10–14 weeks of pregnancy, but this all depends on your particular hospital or antenatal unit.

The dating scan is also important if you are planning to have tests for Down's syndrome (see pages 93–7) and/or spina bifida because if these tests are performed during specific weeks of pregnancy they will be more accurate.

Mum's top tip

I'd suggest you ask your partner or a friend to come with you to the scans, as it can be a very emotional experience. When I went for my dating scan, I thought I was just over ten weeks pregnant. The sonographer told me I was actually 12 weeks pregnant, and what a pleasant surprise that was! I was close to tears when I saw my baby on screen and was so relieved that this pregnancy was going well, particularly because my last pregnancy ended in miscarriage.

HOW ACCURATE IS A DATING SCAN?

The length of your pregnancy and therefore your due date is worked out from the first day of your last period. This is because most women will know when their last monthly period (or LMP) was rather than being able to pinpoint the exact day they conceived (generally assessed as being 12–14 days after the start of their LMP). The point of the dating scan is to ascertain with greater accuracy what stage your baby is at in order to try to reduce the number of women whose labour is induced because their due date was miscalculated.

HOW BIG WILL MY BABY BE AT THIS SCAN?

At 10–14 weeks, your baby will seem very small; in fact she will just look like a blob with a heartbeat jumping around on the screen. At this stage, your baby will be measured from head to bottom – what is referred to as 'crown rump length'. When the foetus is very small, its legs are all curled up, so it is more accurate to measure them from head to bottom.

At around ten weeks, your baby might measure somewhere around 3–4cm (1¼–1½in); at 12 weeks she might measure 5–6cm (2in); and at 13 weeks around 6.5–8cm (2½–3½in). This, of course, is a rough estimate and even at this early stage the size of your baby can vary.

CAN A DATING SCAN SHOW IF I AM HAVING TWINS?

The ultrasound can show whether you are carrying twins or multiples as early as 12 weeks into pregnancy. The sonographer can even identify whether you are carrying identical or fraternal twins by measuring the thickness of the membranes which separate the two amniotic sacs in your uterus. At 12 weeks, it's too early to tell what sex your babies are, however.

Even if there is a history of twins in the family (bearing in mind that the gene often skips a generation), it is likely to come as a complete surprise. Seeing your babies for the first time will be very exciting, even if they just look like two blobs with big heads. Don't be surprised if you go through a multitude of emotions after you discover the news. The sonographers are used to giving new parents unexpected news, so don't fret about what they might think about your own reaction, whether you're in floods of tears or laughing hysterically.

Foetal anomaly scan

The scan for abnormalities, or 'foetal anomaly scan' as it's often referred to, is offered to pregnant women at around 20 weeks of pregnancy in order to check that their baby is developing correctly. At this scan, your baby will be examined closely to ascertain that certain abnormalities do not appear to be present and things are progressing as they should.

In guidelines published by the Royal College of Obstetricians and Gynaecologists, it is stated that around half of all foetal abnormalities will be picked up at the 20-week scan.

This means, of course, that half of all major abnormalities may *not* be seen on screen, and therefore there is still a chance that there may be undiagnosed problems with your baby's development. However, when it comes to detecting certain conditions, this scan is highly effective.

Anencephaly (when a baby's forebrain does not develop), spina bifida, major kidney problems, limb abnormalities and defects of the abdominal wall all have an extremely high chance of being picked up during the 20-week scan. Other conditions, such as congenital heart problems and hydrocephalus (excess fluid on the brain), may also be detected at this stage.

It is at this scan that parents can be told what sex their baby is going to be – if they would like to know, that is. Some parents-to-be prefer to keep it a surprise, waiting until the birth itself.

Antenatal tests

A whole range of antenatal tests may be offered to you (for a fee, in certain cases) to test your baby for certain genetic disorders and congenital conditions.

There are also tests that you can have to check your own health so that you can consider the possible impact it might have on your unborn child. Some of these tests are routine and some need to be requested by you or suggested by your doctor or midwife.

The best known of the different antenatal tests for genetic disorders are probably those for Down's syndrome and for congenital conditions such as spina bifida and anencephaly, but there are many others. Some of these tests carry a small risk of miscarriage, however, which needs to be taken into account.

The important thing to understand is that the tests are not compulsory. You also need to think very carefully about the implications of having certain tests done and what you would do as a result of discovering that your baby was going to have a particular medical condition.

Mum's top tip

Each time I was due to have a routine pregnancy test, I kept dreaming that something was going to happen to my baby. It's just your brain trying to process stuff that you don't think about while you're awake. My advice is to try not to get too stressed about pregnancy tests but talk to your midwife for reassurance. I found it useful to write down any negative thoughts I had, then close the notebook firmly, to shut them out.

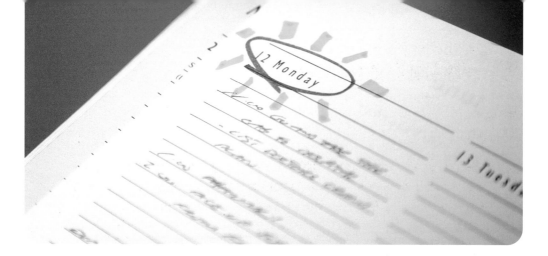

You may want to know so that you can arrange to deliver in a place that has a special care baby unit. You may also want to be able to prepare mentally for such an eventuality. On the other hand, you may want to be able to choose to terminate the pregnancy, should tests show that your baby will be born with a serious medical condition.

Decisions like these are not easy to make, of course, and you should not be put under pressure to take any course of action you are not comfortable with. For every woman and every couple there are specific circumstances to take into account, and making a choice can be affected by many different factors.

Talk to as many people as you can about the implications of certain tests. After an initial chat with your GP or midwife, it may be useful for you to see a counsellor before you decide to go through with certain tests.

Your GP or midwife may be able to recommend a counsellor specializing in the field of antenatal testing. There are also organizations that you can approach for help and support who can put you in touch with other women and couples who have had antenatal testing. (For more information, see Resources, pages 216–17.)

Make sure you and your partner talk about this and share the responsibility for going ahead with any tests you do decide to have. You need to agree on what action you would take in the event of a test result coming back positive.

Screening tests

While screening tests can indicate the risk of your baby having a certain condition such as Down's syndrome, they are not able to tell you categorically that this is the case. Because they are non-invasive and hence carry no risk of miscarriage, this is normally the first step that a pregnant woman will take.

Screening tests include: blood tests that are usually offered at around 16 weeks into your pregnancy; ultrasound scans (see pages 84-9); and the nuchal translucency test for Down's syndrome, (available from about ten weeks of pregnancy – see overleaf).

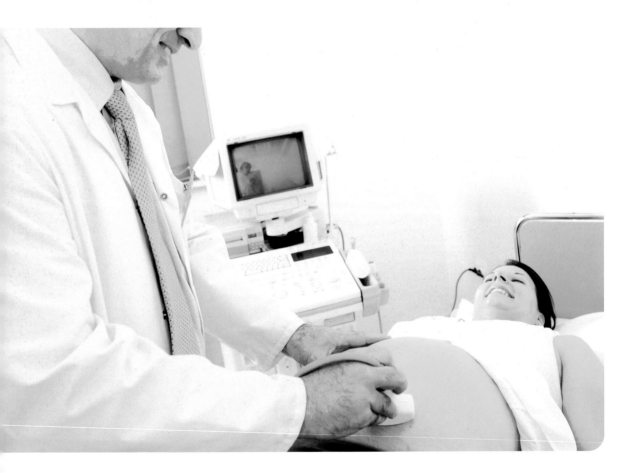

Getting the best antenatal care

Screening tests will tell you your statistical chances of having a baby with a particular condition. If you screen negative, this means that the risk of having a baby with a particular condition is low enough not to be considered a problem, maybe 1 in 300.

In a very small number of cases, couples are told they screen negative and then give birth to a baby with a condition such as Down's syndrome. While very unlikely, it is still feasible that a baby given a screen negative result could be the 1 in 1,000 that is affected by a particular condition.

If you 'screen positive', you are considered to be at a high enough risk to warrant having a diagnostic test. It is important to recognize, however, that screening positive does not mean your baby is definitely affected by a particular condition. Many of the women who screen positive go on to have perfectly healthy babies. These cases are referred to as 'false positives'.

What is Down's syndrome?

Down's syndrome is a life-long, genetic condition that causes delays in learning and development. Affecting around 1 in every 1,000 babies, the condition is caused by the presence of an extra chromosome.

Chromosomes are tiny particles in our bodies that carry the 'blueprint' for all the characteristics we inherit from our parents. There are 23 pairs of chromosomes in each cell, making 46 altogether. We inherit one half of each pair from our fathers and the other half of the pair from our mothers.

In 1959 Professor Jérôme Lejeune, a French geneticist, discovered that some people carry an extra copy of chromosome 21, making 47 chromosomes in all. The condition was named Down's syndrome after the English doctor John Langdon Down, who first noted it in 1866, almost 100 years before the extra chromosome was discovered.

Children with Down's syndrome all share some obvious physical characteristics that doctors and midwives will be looking out for once your baby is born. They will typically have small, upward-slanting eyes with extra skin around them (although this does not affect their eyesight) and a wide-bridged nose.

Down's syndrome babies usually have broad and short hands with a deep crease across the palm. They may also have slightly flatter heads and a pronounced gap between the first and second toe.

A number of screening tests are available to ascertain your risk of having a baby with Down's syndrome, including various blood tests and the nuchal translucency test. If, following screening, you are deemed to be at high risk, then diagnostic testing will be offered to you.

BLOOD TESTS
First trimester
During the first trimester, around weeks 11–14 of pregnancy, you may be offered a blood test that measures levels of the pregnancy hormone HCG (human chorionic gonadotrophin) and PAPP-A (pregnancy-associated plasma protein). If you are carrying a child with Down's syndrome, levels of these two substances in your blood will be raised.

Second trimester
In the second trimester of pregnancy, usually between weeks 15 and 20, your blood may be tested for levels of certain substances known as 'markers'. This test is often referred to as the AFP (alpha-fetoprotein) test, as this protein is one of the markers that is tested.

However, most hospitals provide a test that looks for the presence of two, three or even four different markers, so you may also hear it being referred to as the 'double', 'triple' or even 'quadruple' test. Apart from AFP, the other markers are

HCG, oestriol and inhibin A. If you are carrying a child with Down's syndrome, levels of HCG and inhibin A will be higher in your blood, and AFP and oestriol will be lower.

NUCHAL TRANSLUCENCY TEST

A fairly recent addition to the range of antenatal tests is the nuchal translucency test. This takes place around 10–14 weeks into the pregnancy and combines a blood test with a complex ultrasound scan to establish the level of risk of your baby having Down's syndrome.

Where can I be tested?

The test is only carried out in a certain number of NHS hospitals, unless you opt to have it done privately. Further information can be found from your local midwife.

What happens during the test?

Your baby's heart rate is monitored (babies with a high heart rate are more likely to have Down's syndrome), your age is taken into account (older mothers being more at risk of having a child with the condition), your blood is taken and you are given a detailed, high-resolution abdominal scan.

During the scan, the thin layer of fluid (lying between two folds of skin) at the back of your baby's head is measured. This is because babies with Down's syndrome have a thicker layer of fluid in this part of their bodies. Depending on the quality of the scan, the sonographer may be able to look for other medical conditions such as anencephaly and spina bifida by examining your baby's brain and spine.

When will I get the results?

You will be told your results within about four days. If your test is positive, you may consider further diagnostic tests, such as amniocentisis, to confirm the results.

Diagnostic tests

Diagnostic tests are able to tell you, categorically, whether your baby has a certain condition. They include certain types of ultrasound scans, amniocentesis and chorionic villus sampling. There is a small risk of miscarriage that, for some women, outweighs the benefit of being tested. These tests can also be fairly expensive.

AMNIOCENTESIS

One of the most well-known of the antenatal tests, amniocentesis is routinely offered to women over the age of 35 to establish whether their baby is at risk of having a genetic condition such as Down's syndrome. It can also pick up musculoskeletal disorders such as spina bifida and Duchenne muscular dystrophy, as well as also being able to detect chronic inherited diseases such as cystic fibrosis.

During the test, a tiny sample of amniotic fluid – the fluid that surrounds the foetus in the womb – is removed. This is because the fluid contains cells shed from your baby, which can then be tested for a range of different medical conditions. Usually, this test is carried out when you are around 18 weeks pregnant and you may have to wait another four weeks for the results.

What happens during amniocentesis?

After emptying your bladder, your womb will be scanned, so that the doctor can see the safest place from which to take a sample of amniotic fluid. A long needle is inserted through your tummy into your womb to withdraw a sample of amniotic fluid. The test takes between ten and 30 minutes and afterwards you will be advised to rest for the next 24 hours in order to reduce the risk of miscarriage.

Side effects

It is likely that you will experience mild cramps or pain in the abdomen. However, there are potentially more far-reaching implications of having an amniocentesis and these must be considered before you decide whether to have the test. Potential side effects are as follows:

- The risk of club foot in your baby (the risk being greater the earlier you have the test)
- The needle could injure you or your baby. While this is unlikely, due to the internal guide the ultrasound scan offers your doctor, there is always a small risk of it happening
- If your blood is exposed to that of your baby, this could cause problems if you are rhesus negative and your baby is rhesus positive. Although there is only a tiny possibility of this happening, if there is any doubt you will be offered an injection of 'anti-D', so that you don't react to your baby's red blood cells (For more on rhesus incompatibility, see pages 103-4.)
- A small but real risk of miscarriage (about 1%), which you need to consider carefully before you decide whether or not to proceed.

CHORIONIC VILLUS SAMPLING (CVS)

This is a diagnostic test that is widely available to women over 35 or who have a risk of inherited disorders. It is normally offered in the early stages of pregnancy, from about ten weeks onwards. Because of the risk of miscarriage following this procedure (between 0.5 and 2%), any woman or couple considering this test ought to think very carefully before going ahead with it. It may be best to ask your hospital what their miscarriage rate is following such a procedure.

What happens during CVS?

The test itself is fairly straightforward and takes around 20 minutes to complete. An ultrasound scan is taken to establish where the placenta is lying in your uterus, after which a very fine needle is inserted into your tummy (or occasionally the procedure is carried out through your vagina and cervix) to remove a sample of the placenta.

Your placenta is made up of sections, known chorionic villi, which have been formed by the division of the fertilized egg and which have exactly the same genetic codes or DNA as your baby does. This means that any genetic condition (such as Down's syndrome) in the embryo will be present in the placenta and will be revealed in the sample that is taken. (Please note that this test will not be able to establish whether your baby has spina bifida.)

Special problems in pregnancy

As well as checking that all is well with your baby, your healthcare providers will be keeping a good eye on you too, as occasionally problems can arise.

Gestational diabetes

One problem that they'll be looking out for is a type of diabetes that is unique to pregnancy, occurring in 3–5% of pregnant women. The good news is that it can be managed with a good diet and exercise and, in most cases, goes away after your baby is born, although there is a slightly higher risk of developing diabetes later in life.

At antenatal checks, your urine will be tested for the presence of sugar. If your system is working normally, sugar is turned into stored energy through the insulin produced in the pancreas. If not, then sugar levels rise in the blood. If your GP suspects diabetes, you may need to take a glucose tolerance test. Many antenatal clinics offer this test to all women between weeks 24 and 28, or as early as 16 weeks if diabetes is suspected before then. If you are diagnosed with the

Mum's top tip

I had gestational diabetes with both my first and second children. My first was 8lb 4oz and my second was 9lb 4oz. Both times I had to monitor my blood sugar levels (I was given a special device and shown how to use it). I had to avoid certain foods such as fruit juices, sweets and cakes, but you'll be advised on diet and may possibly be referred to a dietician. As soon as each of my babies was born, I was tested again and my levels were back to normal and no further monitoring was required.

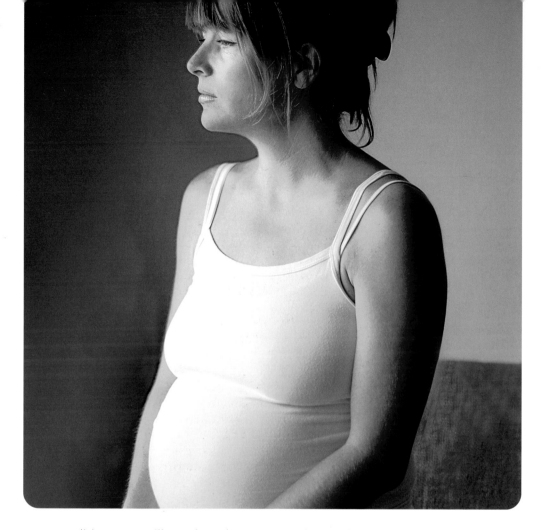

condition, you will need to change your diet and possibly take tablets or insulin injections to control your blood sugar levels. You may be referred to a special antenatal team where you'll be seen by a consultant as well as a midwife and regularly monitored.

DELIVERY OF YOUR BABY

If your diabetes is managed and there are no complications, your pregnancy may be allowed to continue until 39–40 weeks, after which you may need to be induced. Rates of Caesarean section tend to be higher in women with gestational diabetes, but this isn't to say that you can't have a vaginal birth.

POSTNATAL CARE

If you have gestational diabetes, you will be monitored closely after the delivery of your baby, although in most cases insulin levels return to normal after the baby is born. You will also be given a check at six weeks by your diabetes team.

Anaemia during pregnancy

Anaemia is quite common in pregnancy. It arises when the body does not produce enough, or loses too many, red blood cells, which are responsible for carrying oxygen around the body. The oxygen-carrying ability of the red blood cells is measured in grams and referred to as the 'haemoglobin level', which is normally around 12–14g. To maintain levels of red blood cells, the body needs a good supply of iron, as well as folic acid and vitamin B12.

During pregnancy, your body demands more vitamins and especially iron in order to supply both you and your baby. Your blood supply may become diluted during pregnancy and hence your haemoglobin level drops. If it drops below 10g, treatment for anaemia may be given. Your haemoglobin levels will routinely be tested at the beginning of your pregnancy and often in the later stages, especially if you are showing signs of anaemia.

SYMPTOMS OF ANAEMIA

Symptoms of anaemia include feeling very tired, experiencing chest pains or headaches, and occasionally having palpitations or feeling breathless. If you are light-skinned and become anaemic, you will probably look very pale. If you are found to be anaemic you will usually be prescribed an iron supplement.

AVOIDING ANAEMIA

The best way to avoid anaemia is to eat a well-balanced and healthy diet that includes good sources of iron, vitamin B12 and folic acid. Taking a supplement of folic acid is recommended in early pregnancy (and before conception). (For more on the importance of folic acid in pregnancy, and good dietary sources of this, iron and vitamin B12, see pages 42–5.)

TREATMENT FOR ANAEMIA IN A NEWBORN BABY
Babies can also be anaemic, although the condition is often hard to diagnose as there can be no symptoms. If your baby looks pale, or is overly tired, becomes short of breath or very sleepy during feeding, he may be anaemic, although any of these symptoms could be signs of something else entirely. If an older child (or indeed a pregnant woman – see page 54) eats chalk or soil, this can indicate an iron-deficiency problem.

Anaemia is diagnosed with a simple blood test, which will be administered in the maternity unit. The hospital may prescribe iron drops with your baby's feeds. Generally, breastfed babies receive enough iron from their mother's milk, while bottlefed babies will be given an iron-supplemented formula. In severe cases, a baby may need to have blood transfusion, but you will be advised by your doctor and midwife if this is the case.

Rhesus incompatibility

A small percentage of the female population are what is known as rhesus negative. This means they are missing a substance known as the rhesus factor from their blood. In a first pregnancy, when a woman who is rhesus negative is carrying a rhesus-positive baby, it is usually not an issue. However, if blood cells from the baby mix with the mother's blood cells (during delivery or a diagnostic test, for example) then the mother's blood may become 'sensitized'. This means that when the rhesus factor enters the mother's bloodstream, it acts as an antigen and stimulates production of antibodies that will work to attack and destroy the red blood cells of any rhesus-positive baby she becomes pregnant with in the future.

If the father is rhesus negative as well as the mother, there is no risk to the baby as he will be rhesus negative. But if the father is rhesus positive, it could be an issue, and the woman's blood will probably be monitored extremely closely as her pregnancy progresses. If foetal bilirubin is detected in the amniotic fluid, this indicates red blood cells are being destroyed and further treatment may be necessary. In severe cases, an intra-uterine blood transfusion may be required. Usually, after your first delivery, you will be given an injection of 'anti-D' to protect you for future pregnancies. If you are concerned about any of these issues, talk to your GP about it.

Pre-eclampsia

Pre-eclampsia, or pregnancy-induced hypertension, is thought to occur among 8–10% of pregnant women, 85% of whom are pregnant for the first time. It is the most common form of maternal death in the UK, killing around ten women a year. It also leads to the death of about 1,000 babies a year.

WHAT ARE THE SYMPTOMS?

Pre-eclampsia is characterized by high blood pressure, swelling of the hands and feet, and protein in the urine. Other symptoms include persistent headaches, blurred vision and flashing lights, and abdominal pain on the right side of the body below the ribcage. Many women suffering from pre-eclampsia feel fine and only learn of the condition when their blood pressure is found to be high. Pre-eclampsia typically occurs after 20 weeks gestation, but it can occur earlier.

AM I AT RISK?

Pre-eclampsia can affect anyone, but those more at risk are mothers over 40, teenage mothers, or those who have diabetes, a history of high blood pressure, kidney or rheumatology problems.

WHAT IS THE TREATMENT?

The causes of pre-eclampsia are uncertain, but research suggests it may be linked to an immune reaction by the mother to the foetus or the placenta. Pre-eclampsia is often hereditary. Women suffering from it are advised to rest or take tablets to reduce their blood pressure. Delivery of the baby is the only cure and induction or a Caesarean section may be performed if the mother is severely affected. Your baby may have to be delivered before term (37 weeks). Pre-eclampsia subsides within about 48 hours of the baby being delivered. If early pre-eclampsia is detected, you may be advised to have complete bed rest and take blood pressure tablets. Sometimes, hospitalization may be required.

IS THERE ANYTHING I CAN DO?
Stress causes blood pressure to rise, so try to eliminate anything stressful from your life. Eat plenty of fresh fruit and vegetables, cut down on salt and fat in your diet and drink lots of water. Attend every check-up, as your midwife or GP will check your blood pressure and test your urine for high levels of protein.

Eclampsia

Pre-eclampsia can develop into eclampsia, which is a rare but serious condition, characterized by seizures and possibly coma. Urgent delivery of the baby is required and the mother will be treated with drugs to stop the seizures.

WILL I HAVE PRE-ECLAMPSIA AGAIN WITH MY NEXT PREGNANCY?
If your first pregnancy was normal (apart from the pre-eclampsia), your risk of developing it again with your next pregnancy is very low. If, however, there are other factors such as a family history of high blood pressure, you are overweight or an older mother, you will probably be monitored closely during your next pregnancy, just to be on the safe side. By contrast, a study in Scotland has revealed that 1 in 150 women whose blood pressure had been entirely normal during their first pregnancy suffered from pre-eclampsia in a second pregnancy. Hence it is a condition that is not easy to predict.

Mum's top tip

Don't get too stressed about pre-eclampsia. I had all the usual antenatal checks on blood pressure and urine during my pregnancy, but because I had a history of pre-eclampsia, I was also given more frequent ultrasound scans to check on my baby's growth, tests to check that my kidneys were working well and that my blood-clotting function was good, and Doppler scans to make sure that my baby was getting a good supply of blood through the placenta. I actually found it all very reassuring and my baby was fine.

Losing a baby

Miscarriage refers to when a pregnancy terminates before the sixth month and is estimated to occur in about 10-20% of pregnancies. It is hard to give an exact figure because many women miscarry before they even realize they are pregnant, simply assuming it was a very heavy period.

The majority of miscarriages happen in the first three months of pregnancy. At least half of all miscarriages which occur in the first trimester are caused by chromosomal abnormalities that prevent the foetus from developing normally. Later miscarriage, usually in the second trimester, is more likely to be a result of the placenta not functioning properly.

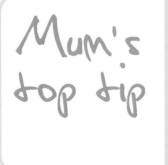

Mum's top tip

I had a miscarriage at 11 weeks and have just found out I'm pregnant again. It can be very helpful to talk to other people who have gone through a similar experience, so if you feel you need to talk to someone about your loss, but don't know who to talk to, contact the Miscarriage Association. Just try to remember that this happens to one in every five pregnancies. It's a very difficult time, but you will gradually start to feel better.

The symptoms of miscarriage are vaginal bleeding accompanied by lower backache and severe stomach cramps, a bit like period pain. Lots of women experience vaginal bleeding in early pregnancy and go on to have a normal pregnancy and healthy baby. Experts are not sure why this happens, but it affects roughly one in five women.

Once the uterus starts to expel the foetus, there is little that can be done to save it. An ultrasound will probably be required to establish what stage you are at, or if you are miscarrying at all. You will either have an external ultrasound scan in which a transducer (looking a bit like a microphone) is placed on your lower abdomen, or if the pregnancy is very early, you may have to have an internal ultrasound in which a probe is inserted into your vagina. Neither procedure hurts.

COMPLETE MISCARRIAGE

A complete miscarriage occurs where the uterus expels the foetus and placenta entirely, and an ultrasound scan shows that the uterus is entirely empty.

MISSED MISCARRIAGE

A missed miscarriage is where the foetus and placenta die but remain in the mother's womb for some time before being expelled. There might be very minor symptoms such as a brownish discharge. An ultrasound can check whether the foetus's heart has stopped beating, or look for an empty sac inside the uterus.

INCOMPLETE MISCARRIAGE

An incomplete miscarriage occurs where a miscarriage happens but some of the products of conception are left inside the mother.

What is the treatment for miscarriage?

If you start to bleed at any time during the second or third trimester, call your maternity unit and go there as soon as possible. If you are bleeding in your first trimester, call your doctor and stop any sexual activities and exercise. Your doctor will probably refer you to an early pregnancy unit at the hospital, or the gynaecological department, and you will be given an ultrasound to see whether a miscarriage is imminent.

If a miscarriage is inevitable, there is little doctors can do to stop it. You may be given the option to see if the pregnancy is expelled from your body naturally over the next few days. Most women are offered a procedure known as ERPC (evacuation of retained products of conception), a minor operation conducted under general anaesthetic, to clean out the uterus. It involves dilating the cervix and scraping tissue away from the lining of the uterus.

Incompetent cervix

Experts believe that in 20–25% of cases of late miscarriage, in the second trimester, an incompetent cervix is the cause. This is a condition in which the cervix opens under the pressure of the growing baby, possibly leading to miscarriage or premature delivery. Late miscarriage can also be caused by a genetically weak cervix, damage following a previous difficult birth, previous surgery on the cervix, laser therapy or a cone biopsy for cervical cancer.

HOW WILL I KNOW IF I HAVE AN INCOMPETENT CERVIX?
It is usually diagnosed if you have previously had a miscarriage in your second trimester, or it is noticed during an internal examination or ultrasound scan.

WHAT IS THE TREATMENT?
The treatment for an incompetent cervix is to sew it closed to reinforce it. The procedure is usually performed between 12 and 16 weeks of pregnancy to prevent any problems when you go into labour. The stitches are removed before the estimated delivery date, or as labour starts. The chances of carrying a baby to term following this procedure are very good.

Getting the best antenatal care

Ectopic pregnancy

This is a serious condition in which the pregnancy develops outside the womb, usually in the fallopian tubes. An ectopic pregnancy is not capable of surviving and will normally spontaneously miscarry. The most common symptoms are vaginal bleeding, abdominal pain, which can be quite severe, and sometimes shoulder or rectal pain. An ectopic pregnancy can be life-threatening if it ruptures and causes internal bleeding, so if you experience unusual vaginal bleeding or abdominal pain, contact your GP or midwife at once.

WHAT ARE THE SYMPTOMS?
Abdominal bleeding – often dark and watery and sometimes described as looking like prune juice, abdominal pain, pain when urinating, sickness, diarrhoea and feeling faint.

CAN ANYONE EXPERIENCE AN ECTOPIC PREGNANCY?
Any woman can experience an ectopic pregnancy, but you are more at risk if you have endometriosis, pelvic inflammatory disease, if you are over 35 or you smoke.

WHAT IS THE TREATMENT?
If an ectopic pregnancy is suspected, a laparoscopy (keyhole surgery) can be performed to remove it. If the pregnancy is not too far advanced, a relatively new medical treatment known as methotrexate may be used. Administered by injection, this stops the growth of rapidly dividing cells and induces miscarriage.

WHAT HAPPENS FOLLOWING TEATMENT?
If you take methotrexate, you are likely to bleed for one to two weeks, although some women report bleeding and spotting for up to six weeks. Your periods will probably restart around 6–10 weeks following surgery or four weeks after taking methotrexate.

HOW LONG WILL IT TAKE TO GET PREGNANT AGAIN?
The use of methotrexate does not reduce your chances of getting pregnant in the future and 65% of women will become pregnant within 18 months of trying. Your chances are possibly higher than if the pregnancy is removed surgically, which can cause scarring around the fallopian tube.

Planning for the birth

Childbirth preparation classes

It's important to attend a childbirth preparation class, if you can. Many antenatal classes are available and you should decide which course suits you best.

Hospitals tend to run their own classes. As well as providing information about pregnancy, labour and birth, the person taking the class may also talk through topics such as hospital policy and where to park your car, and you may be taken on a tour of the labour ward. The advantage of these classes is that they are generally free, but if you are planning a home delivery, or are not going to that particular hospital to give birth, they may not be as relevant to you.

Private classes, run by organizations such as the National Childbirth Trust (see Resources, pages 216–17, for contact details), may focus on labour and pain relief, in addition to other options such as natural childbirth (see pages 116–17). You will have to pay for these sessions and ensure you book early as they tend to get booked up quickly.

Some GP surgeries may also have classes, so do ask if your surgery runs them. You may prefer to be in a big class where you and your partner can meet lots of other parents-to-be, but equally you can pay for small, private sessions where you're the only couple.

Questions to ask at the classes

- How do I know when I'm in labour?
- What do I do if my waters have broken?
- (For the birth partner) How can I help?
- What should I pack for labour and birth?
- How long will I need to stay in hospital after the birth?
- What different methods of pain relief are available?
- Where can I get advice on breastfeeding?

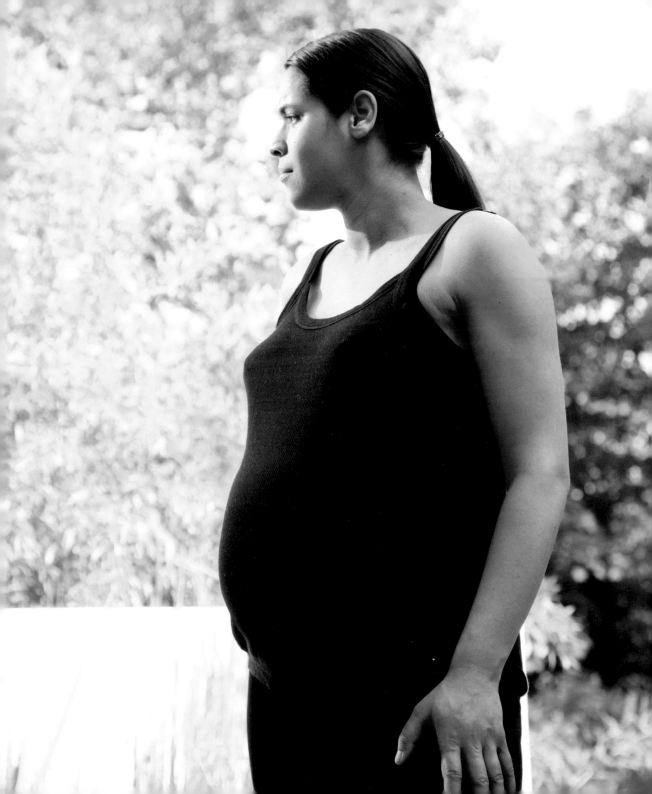

Birth plans

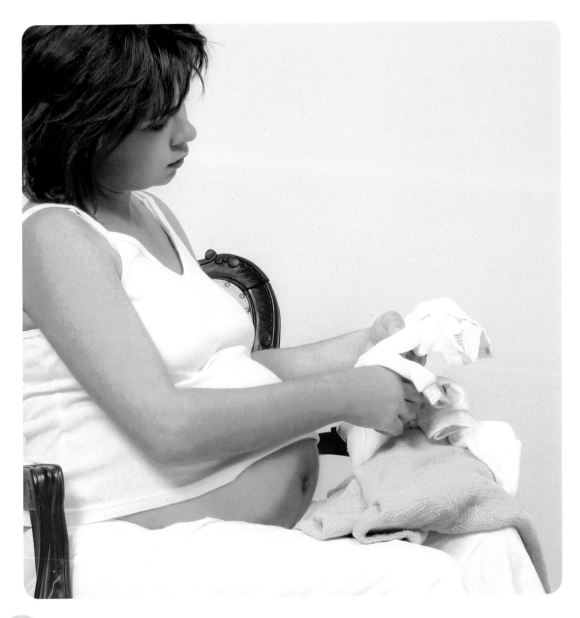

A birth plan is a plan you draw up to express how you would like things to happen during your labour. It helps you to become an active participant in the birth, rather than feeling left out of any decisions that might be taken on your behalf.

It is increasingly common, these days, for women (and their partners) to want to take a more active role in their birthing experience. Doctors and midwives generally acknowledge this need by encouraging you to draw up a plan. The birth plan is not a legal document, but it does allow the parents-to-be to express their expectations and hopes for the birth. A plan like this is also helpful for midwives and doctors.

It is in your birth plan that you can express your desire for things such as: the number of birth partners you want to be there; how long you want to remain in hospital; if you would like to use a birthing pool; and the type of pain relief, if any, that you want. You may also like to write down how you feel about the necessity for forceps or an episiotomy.

Having read through the plan, your midwife might address any unrealistic expectations raised by it (more likely if you are a first-time mum), talking through what is and isn't possible. But do remember that a birth plan is just that, a plan, and although you may want your baby's birth to happen in a certain way, sometimes it will not be in the best interests of you or your baby to follow the course of action requested by you. Having expressed your preferences, the important thing is to remain flexible and prepared to change your mind.

Top tips for writing your birth plan

Go to all your antenatal classes to find out exactly what is involved at each stage of labour and the options for pain relief. Talk to friends who have given birth about their experiences to help you make up your mind about the kind of birth you would like. Here are some questions to ask yourself when writing your plan.

SUPPORT
Who do you want with you at the birth and who don't you want? Sometimes relatives and friends can turn up unexpectedly. thinking they can help. If you suspect this might happen, let your midwife know that she can send them away.

WHERE
Do you want to give birth in hospital or at home? Are you considering a birthing suite or having a water birth (see pages 122–3)? Do you want a home birth or a hospital birth? If you want a home birth, discuss this with your midwife or GP first so that they can assess whether this is feasible in your case.

EQUIPMENT
Do you want a birthing stool, or birthing ball? Do you have your own TENS machine or do you plan to hire one (see page 119)?

INDUCTION
Are you prepared for the fact you might have to be induced (see pages 140–2)?

POSITIONS YOU WANT TO BE IN FOR LABOUR
Would you prefer to have an active labour where you move from position to position, or do you want to remain lying down? (For more on positions in labour, see pages 176–7.)

PAIN RELIEF
Do you want to avoid pain relief, or will you keep your options open in case the discomfort gets too much? It is up to you whether you want drugs or not, and you can change your mind if things become unbearable. If you are keen to have an

top tips

epidural (see pages 182–3), make sure you tell your midwife when you are admitted so that arrangements can be made.

EPISIOTOMY
Most women want to avoid an episiotomy (see pages 188–91) unless it is absolutely necessary. Discuss this with your midwife.

CAESAREAN SECTION
Do you want to try everything you can before a Caesarean is considered? If you do have a Caesarean (see pages 130–33), does your partner want to be in theatre with you?

YOUR BABY
Do you want your baby to be monitored with a foetal heart monitor, or would you prefer not, unless necessary? Would you like the midwife to tell you the sex of your baby or would you and your partner like to find out for yourselves? Would you like your baby delivered onto your abdomen? Will your partner cut the cord, or would you prefer one of the medical team to do it? Would you prefer your baby to be cleaned up before being given to you? Do you want to try to breastfeed straight away?

AFTER THE BIRTH
Do you want to deliver the placenta naturally or use drugs to encourage delivery? Do you want your baby to be given vitamin K (see pages 209–10)?

Mum's top tip

I strongly recommend that you make a birth plan. The important things to think about are: who you'd like to be your birth partner; your choice of pain relief; and if you want the baby placed straight onto your tummy. Note any religious requirements and if you want to breastfeed straight away. To be honest, everything else becomes of little consequence when you're in labour and you may well change your mind about what's in your birth plan.

top tips

Natural birth

If you plan to have as natural a birth as possible, the right breathing technique will help you achieve this, as long, slow breaths in and out will relax you and help you to focus. Breathing properly means that your muscles will relax rather than stiffen up, which will help to ease the pain of contractions. For more on breathing techniques during labour, see pages 144–5.

Lots of women make it through labour without any pain relief, or just relying on gas and air. If you do have medication for pain relief, you shouldn't feel guilty or that you have failed in some way. Every woman reacts to pain differently, so whatever helps you get through labour, be it screaming at the top of your voice or cramming in as many drugs as possible, is entirely up to you and your midwife.

Planning for a natural birth

Babies, labour and birth are unpredictable, and even the best-laid plans can take unexpected twists and turns. (For a more detailed look at the different stages of labour, see pages 170–5.)

Staying at home for as long as you can will help your chances of having a natural birth, as a hospital environment can make you feel tense, thus slowing down the birthing process. Using a TENS machine and gas and air (see overleaf) can be a good alternative to drugs for pain relief and many women find them useful.

Adopting different positions can aid a natural birth, most of which use gravity to help the baby move down the birth canal. Standing, squatting or kneeling while upright can all be beneficial, although you may need some physical support to achieve them. (For more advice on positions in labour, see pages 176–7.)

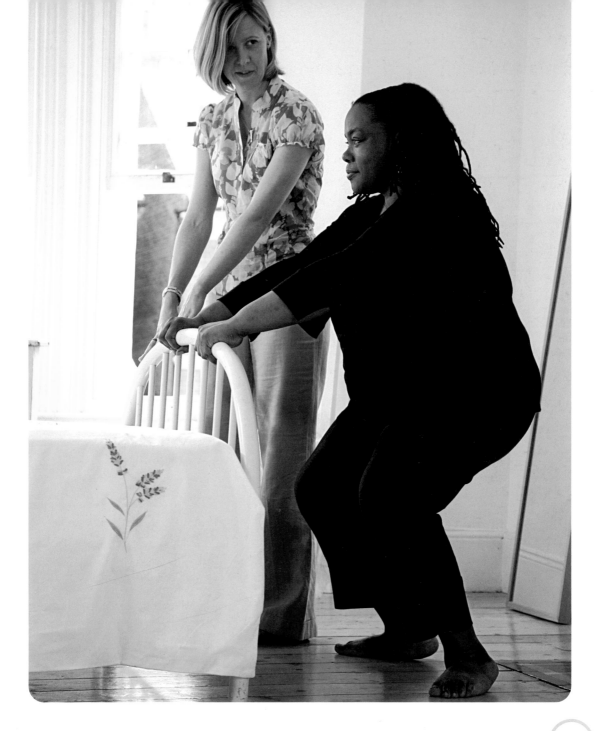

Home birth

Many women choose to have their babies in the familiar surroundings of their home, and statistics show that home births in the UK have risen by 7% in recent years. If you are perfectly healthy or had a straightforward delivery of a previous baby, there should be no reason why you can't have your baby at home, although of course each pregnancy is different and you should seek medical advice beforehand.

The main advantages of a home birth are that you are in relaxed and comfortable surroundings, and you have one-on-one care from your midwife. You'll have the same midwife, or midwife team, throughout labour and birth, and they won't go off shift as they do in hospital. Home birth is great for your partner and any children you have already as they can stay with you as you wish. After your baby is born, providing everything runs smoothly, you will be left with your partner and new baby to bond, breastfeed and recover in the comfort of your own home. With home births, medical intervention is much less likely and you are usually able to stick more closely to your birth plan.

The disadvantages of a home birth are that although it is very rare that problems occur, it can still happen. If the delivery is proving difficult, or the baby has breathing difficulties once born, you may have to go to hospital. Births can also be pretty messy and loud, so any children you do have will have to be warned, or taken to stay elsewhere during the labour.

Pain relief during a home birth

You can't have an epidural in a home birth as this has to be administered by an anaesthetist, but a variety of other options are available, including the ones listed below (For more details about natural pain relief, see pages 178–9.)

TENS MACHINE
TENS stands for 'transcutaneous electrical nerve stimulation', and the machine, attached by electrodes to your skin, works by sending small electrical impulses into your body with every contraction, blocking the pain and encouraging your body to release endorphins, which act as natural painkillers.

A TENS machine can be hired before you go into labour. Being small and portable, it is ideal for a home birth as it can be used anywhere except in a birthing pool. Ask your midwife or doctor about hiring one.

GAS AND AIR (ENTONOX)
Your midwife will bring portable canisters of gas and air (also known as entonox) with her if you think you will need them. (For more on this form of pain relief, see page 180.)

PETHIDINE AND MEPTAZINOL
Some midwives use these pain relief drugs (see page 182) at a home birth, although they tend to prefer not to because the drugs make the baby drowsy and hence in need of closer monitoring. Ask your midwife which pain relief drugs she uses.

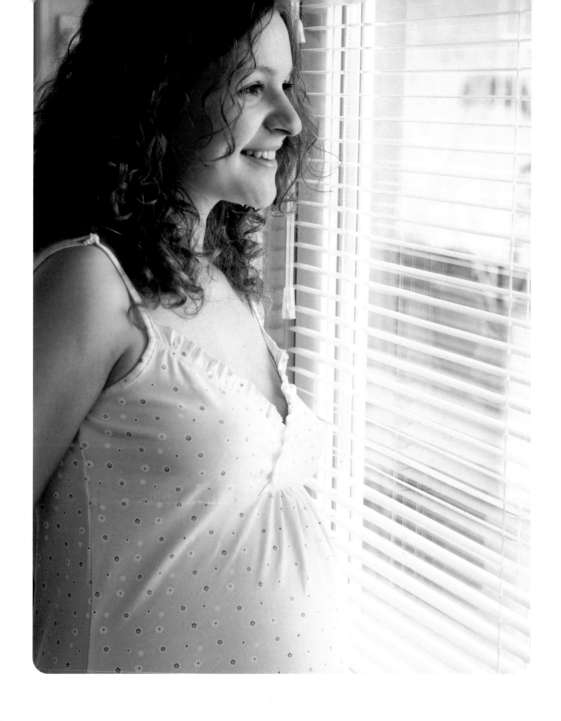

Planning for the birth

Which midwives will attend a home birth?

The number of midwives available to attend homebirths will depend on the area in which you live, the hospital to which you are assigned, and the demand on services at the time you go into labour.

Some women opt for an independent midwife for their home birth, which means they have to pay but are guaranteed the midwife of their choice once they go into labour. Independent midwives usually have the philosophy of one mother, one baby, so you'll see the same midwife throughout your pregnancy – at all antenatal checks as well as during labour and birth. (For more information about independent midwives, see pages 75.)

If you opt to have a home birth, you will contact your midwife to join you when your contractions are coming consistently every 15 minutes (or faster) and when they last for a good minute or so. Your midwife, once she has established that you are in labour, will come to your house to help you give birth.

Your midwife will be able to deal with a normal delivery (and can provide you with pain-relieving drugs such as entonox and pethidine – see the previous page). She will be equipped with resuscitation and intravenous equipment just in case, but if there was a serious problem, you would be transferred to hospital immediately. Your midwife will assess every home birth for its suitability as it progresses, recommending a hospital delivery if that looks to be the safer option. If you do need to be transported to hospital, due to a complication during a home birth, your midwife will be able to arrange this.

Water birth

Giving birth in water can create a soothing environment and provide natural pain relief for you, as well as a comfortable environment for your baby to be born into.

Most hospitals have birthing pools, although they may only have one or two, and therefore work on a first come, first served basis. If you are having your baby at home you can hire a birthing pool for home use. Getting into a bath after a long day can clear your mind and relax your body; having a water birth works in much the same way.

Benefits of a water birth

RELAXATION
Relaxing in water is a great form of pain relief. Water can't take the pain away, but it can help you to feel more relaxed and able to cope with contractions. In water your heart rate slows and your blood pressure is lowered, reducing feelings of tension and stress. Studies show that relaxing in water also helps your body to release endorphins, which act as natural painkillers.

MOBILITY
Water can support the weight of many labour positions, such as squatting or kneeling on all fours, which are quite tricky to sustain on dry land. Water can also support the weight of your body, making it easier to move around.

A SPECIAL ENVIRONMENT
The water surrounding you can help you feel as though you are in your own private world – a special place just for giving birth. Some pools are big enough for your partner to get in with you.

A NATURAL BIRTH

Water can help to speed up labour, by stimulating the production of oxytocin, which can bring on more powerful contractions and faster dilation of the cervix. It therefore reduces the need for medical intervention or pain relief drugs. It can also soften your perineum, reducing the need for an episiotomy (see pages 188–91).

YOUR BABY

Healthy newborn babies are born with a 'dive' reflex, which stops them from taking breaths for a few seconds after the birth. Oxygen is provided for them through the placenta so they can safely be delivered into the water, taking their first breath once they're lifted out.

When a water birth isn't possible

● Not all maternity units have a birthing pool, and, if they do, and it is in use, you may not be able to use it. (Ask your maternity unit about its birthing pool facilities.)

● There are certain medical conditions where a water birth is not advisable – for example, if you are carrying twins or your baby is breech. Discuss this with your GP or midwife.

● If you have had an epidural or been given pethidine, you will not be able to use the birthing pool.

● You have to be at least 37 weeks pregnant to use a birthing pool because premature babies are still too undeveloped to be born into water.

HypnoBirthing

It sounds like the answer to the prayers of countless mums-to-be: giving birth with hugely reduced pain but without the need for invasive drugs for pain relief.

That's the promise of HypnoBirthing, a system of hypnotherapy based on breathing and relaxation techniques which claims not only to significantly reduce labour pain, but to induce such a state of calm that women actually welcome each contraction.

And if you feel sceptical about such claims, so much the better. According to advocates of HypnoBirthing, the more cynical you are, the more likely you will be to benefit from the techniques.

Mum's top tip

I recommend trying HypnoBirthing. For me, it was a really effective way of preparing for birth. I listened to a CD while relaxing in the bath or going to sleep. It helped me with breathing techniques and taught me to visualize restful, positive things. I also used a TENS machine during labour, which some people say don't work but I thought it was great! Getting into a birthing pool between contractions was very relaxing too.

That's not all that HypnoBirthing promises. Its fans say it can also reduce the need for technological assistance, significantly shorten labour, encourage breech babies to assume the correct position, and even aid postnatal recovery.

Reducing fear-tension-pain

HypnoBirthing teaches women self-hypnosis techniques, including simple relaxation and breathing methods. This is supposed to eliminate fear-induced stress and pain during birth. This 'fear-tension-pain' syndrome occurs, so the thinking goes, when a woman is frightened of giving birth. Fear makes her muscles tense up, causing her to fight against her body and nature, which would otherwise do most of the work to push the baby out. So labour becomes more difficult or grinds to a halt, making the mother even more distressed. Thus a cycle of fear, tension and pain is created.

HypnoBirthing aims to stop this cycle before it begins and keep the woman confident and calm throughout labour and birth. One of the ways it seeks to do this is through teaching simple self-hypnosis, although it stresses that women will be alert and fully in control throughout the birth.

Contact the HypnoBirthing Centre for more information (see Resources, pages 216–17, for contact details) and visit a practitioner to find out more. Bear in mind that it would be best to arrange this well in advance of your due date.

Hospital birth

Hospitals and maternity units are now paying more attention to what women want, so you are more likely to give birth in the way that you wish. Most hospitals have birthing pools, CD players for your music and private rooms where you can deliver your baby in peace. Hospitals might not be as familiar as home, but if you surround yourself with items that help you to feel relaxed and comfortable, you will feel more in control at the birth.

If you attend antenatal classes at your hospital, you may be given a tour of the maternity ward; if not, it might be worth asking at your next antenatal appointment whether you can be shown around. It's worth familiarizing yourself with where the maternity ward is (you might need to get there in a hurry!) and what the rooms are like. Depending on your hospital, you may have a private bathroom or access to a birthing pool for a water birth.

As soon as you are admitted to the maternity unit, a midwife will ask you about your labour so far, how many contractions you are having, and the distance they are apart. Make a note of when or if your waters have broken and whether you are feeling pain anywhere else, such as in your lower back. Your midwife will examine you to see how dilated your cervix is and you may have to wear a foetal monitor to check your baby's heartbeat. Don't forget to bring your notes with you when you are admitted, as these show the details of your pregnancy so far.

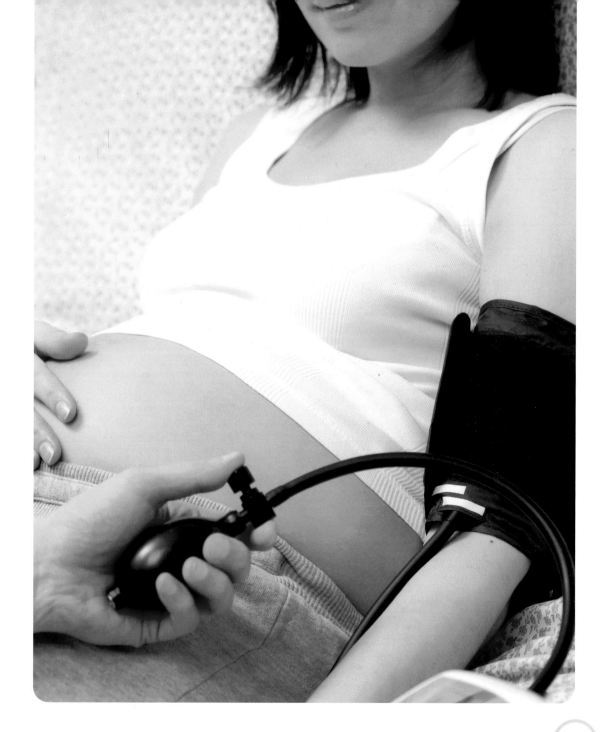

How long am I likely to stay in hospital?

How long you stay in hospital all depends on what kind of birth you have and the health of you and your baby following delivery.

If you have a straightforward vaginal birth with no complications, you might be able to go home the same day or the day after you give birth, providing the midwives are happy that your baby is feeding well. Although you are probably desperate to go home, it's not a bad thing if you have to stay a day or two after the birth because the midwives will help you to establish breast- or bottle-feeding and will show you useful techniques such as how to give your baby a bath and how to wind her properly.

If you have had a Caesarean section, you won't be as mobile after the birth and you should expect to stay in hospital for at least five days. Your blood pressure will be checked and also your abdominal scar to make sure you are healing properly. While the stay in hospital may be frustrating, it can give you time to learn how to care for your baby while help is on hand and while your body heals.

Mum's top tip

I had my first baby in a busy, over-stretched hospital but the care I received was second to none. My advice is to ask loads of questions! The ward was busy but the midwives couldn't have been more helpful. I didn't have a clue about how to breastfeed or give my baby a bath – they showed me how. I felt so secure, surrounded by such expertise, I almost didn't want to leave!

Hospital birth – the pros

- In an emergency situation, you and your baby can be helped immediately.
- You don't have to look after your other children.
- You may be able to stay for a couple of days to recover.
- You will get help with breastfeeding.
- You may get help with aspects of your baby's care, such as how to bathe her.
- You will be able to get a bit of rest (although bear in mind that hospitals are not hotels – they are generally hot, bright and noisy!).
- You will meet lots of other mums, all of whom have just been through what you have, and probably live in the same area as you.

Hospital birth – the cons

- Shifts change daily, so the same midwives may not treat you throughout your stay.
- You are more likely to have medical intervention, such as a Caesarean, if something does go wrong, and you may be given an episiotomy to ease delivery.
- If you live far away from the hospital, bear in mind you have to travel to get there and this can be tricky if contractions are very painful, or your baby is coming quickly.
- Hospital births can mean mixed emotions for your partner. On the plus side, you will be in the safe hands of the hospital staff, which will put him at ease, but he may feel like a spare part, especially if you are in a lot of pain.
- You can't be a proper family straight away, although some hospitals allow partners to stay overnight.

Caesarean section

An elective Caesarean is when the decision to have a Caesarean section is made before labour starts. It's useful to know about the procedure, so that if you do have one you know what to expect.

The most common reasons for your baby to be born this way are if he is breech, his head is too big to pass through your pelvis, or if you are pregnant with twins or multiples. You may need a Caesarean if you suffer from certain medical conditions such as placenta praevia (in which the placenta lies over the cervix). If you have had a Caesarean previously, you may need another, because there is a small risk of uterine rupture when you go into labour.

Elective Caesareans are often carried out under a spinal block or epidural. This means you will be conscious throughout the procedure and will be able to hold your baby as soon as he is born. Your birth partner can be present if he or she wishes, and will have to wear a hospital gown throughout. A screen will be put up so that you cannot see what the surgeon is doing. Often this is taken down when the baby is lifted out, so you can witness the moment your baby enters the world, as in a vaginal birth.

You will have to have a catheter (a small tube for draining urine) fitted if you have a Caesarean so your bladder can be emptied, preventing it getting in the surgeon's way. The catheter is fitted while the spinal block is in place, so you won't feel a thing.

What happens during a Caesarean?

Once you have been injected with the anaesthetic, the effects will be almost immediate. You will be sprayed with an ice-cold spray to confirm the anaesthetic is working. You may feel a tingling sensation in the lower part of your body, and your legs will start to feel heavy. There will be no feeling from your bump downwards and you will feel no pain. Once the surgeon is certain the anaesthetic is working, an incision will be made in your lower abdomen. (Most hospitals these days favour a horizontal 'bikini' cut, just below the top of your pubic hair. You may need to be shaved before the procedure.) A second incision is then made in your uterus and the amniotic sac is opened and drained.

Your baby will be pulled out of your stomach gently, either manually or by using forceps. His airways will be cleared and you will probably hear his first cry. If the screen has been taken down, you will be able to see your baby entering the world. As in a vaginal delivery, the cord will be clamped and cut, and the surgeon will do a quick routine check on your baby, while the placenta is being removed.

Your baby will be handed to you, and while you coo over how amazing he is, you will be stitched up – but you will hardly notice a thing, as your thoughts will be on your brand new baby!

How do I prepare myself for a Caesarean?

You will be told not to eat or drink for a number of hours before the procedure, and you might need an overnight stay in the hospital beforehand. A consent form needs to be signed before the operation, and you will be talked through the procedure by someone on the medical team.

Now is the time to ask any questions, flagging up any needs and requests you might have. Do you want to find out the baby's sex yourself, for example, or do you want to be told? Do you want to try to breastfeed straight away? Your midwife should be able to help you with any concerns.

Are there other types of Caesarean?

Emergency and 'crash' Caesareans won't be planned, tending to take place once labour has started.

An emergency Caesarean usually takes place if your baby is showing signs of distress or if labour is progressing very slowly. An epidural can still be used in an emergency, but your partner may not be allowed to be present at the operation.

A crash Caesarean occurs when your baby needs to be delivered immediately – if your baby is showing severe signs of distress, for instance, or if there are signs of placental abruption or a prolapsed cord. You will probably need a general anaesthetic.

Recovery after a Caesarean

Most women will be able to walk again (if slowly and perhaps painfully), the day after they have had a Caesarean. The best thing to do is attempt walking as soon as you can. Each time you walk it will be less painful than before and the strength will slowly return to your lower body. It is also advisable to be mobile to help prevent blood clots forming and you will probably be given special socks or tights to wear during your hospital stay. You will also be given pain relief to help with the initial stages of recovery.

How you will feel emotionally

You may feel disappointed after having a Caesarean, especially if you didn't even go into labour (if you had an elective Caesarean for a medical reason, for example). You may feel as if you've missed out on the birth experience because your baby didn't come into the world via the traditional route. However, as studies show, there is no difference in the bonding process between mums and babies born vaginally and mums and babies born by Caesarean section.

It can also be tough recovering from a major operation at the same time as looking after a newborn baby, and you may feel overwhelmed by it all. Ensure that any visitors know that you need time to recover, and try to keep visits to a minimum.

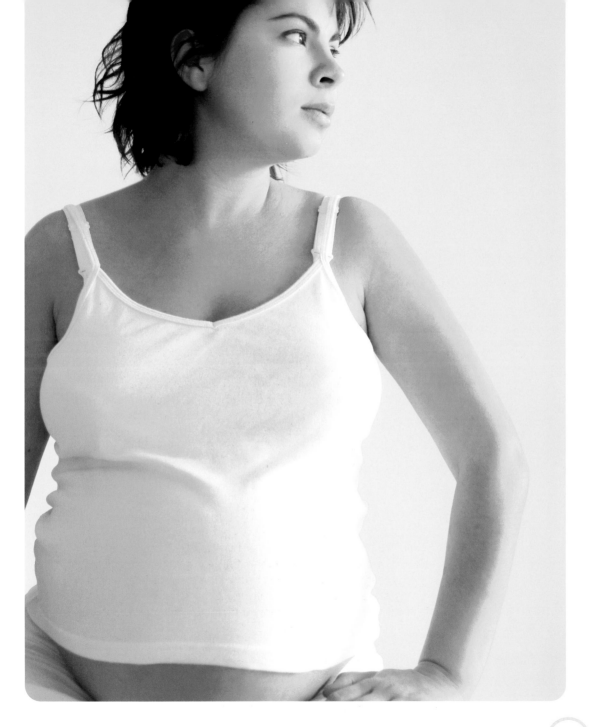

Premature labour and birth

If your baby is born before the end of week 37, she will be considered premature. Some premature babies need no assistance after birth, while others need help to breathe. Your baby's lungs are one of the last organs to fully develop in the womb because she doesn't need to use them until she's born and starts breathing air. This is why premature babies sometimes have breathing problems and have to be transferred to a special care baby unit (SCBU) for a time.

When and why does premature labour occur?

Premature labour is more likely to occur if:

- You have pre-eclampsia (see pages 104–5) or renal disease

- The placenta is not working properly, and your baby stops growing and developing

- There is cord prolapse, placental abruption (premature separation of the placenta) or antepartum haemorrhage (bleeding before term)

- You're showing signs of eclampsia (see page 105)

- You are carrying twins or multiples, because there is no room left in the uterus for the babies to reach full term

- You have had a previous pre-term labour with another baby

- You are younger than 17 or older than 35.

Can premature labour be stopped?

If your medical team think it is safer to stop you going into pre-term labour and better to let your baby grow for as long as she can, they may give you medication to stop labour. Premature babies born between 34 and 37 weeks have a very good chance of surviving, but if your labour starts before 34 weeks you may be given medication to delay labour until you reach at least 34 weeks. You'll have to stay in hospital to be monitored and will need lots of rest.

Premature babies can often be born by normal vaginal birth, but depending on the circumstances, you may need medical assistance. When you arrive at the maternity ward, you will be assessed by the medical team who will advise you on how best to proceed. Sometimes it is safer for babies to be born by Caesarean section if they are very premature, to avoid any of the complications that can happen with a vaginal birth.

How do I know if I am in premature labour?

Symptoms of premature labour will be similar to those of full-term labour, so you may experience any one or all of the following:

- Vaginal bleeding or spotting
- An increase in vaginal discharge
- Discharge that looks watery or mucus-like (this could be a 'show' – see page 161)
- Menstrual-like cramping, lower abdominal pain and more than four contractions in one hour
- Pressure in your pelvic area
- Lower back pain

Contact your midwife or maternity unit immediately if any of these symptoms occur.

The special care baby unit

Your baby may be placed in an incubator so that she can be carefully monitored and the right environment maintained. Seeing her surrounded by wires and beeping equipment can be very distressing, but the special care baby unit (SCBU) is the best place for her. She will be given expert care and there is a high ratio of carers to babies.

You will be encouraged to spend lots of time making contact and interacting with your baby even while she is in the incubator. As there are generally no restrictions on visiting times (although this will depend on your SCBU), you will be able to stay with her as long as you want. Specially trained staff will help you with expressing milk and feeding your baby. They can also lend a hand with changing nappies and giving her a bath.

If your baby is in an incubator or has a feeding tube, you may not be able to hold her all the time, of course, but the midwives can assist you if your baby is well enough. You will also be encouraged to touch her as much as possible and also to talk to her so she knows you are there.

It can be upsetting for you to leave your baby in the SCBU, especially if you have to go home. The staff are specially trained to help you if you feel low, and there will be other parents who are in the same situation as you, who you can talk to if it helps.

Most premature babies are admitted to an intensive care room, where they will be observed and assessed. They will then move into other rooms as their condition improves and they are able to breathe on their own or are doing well with feeding.

Going home

Your baby will stay in the special care baby unit until she can feed and breathe properly, and weighs at least 2kg (4lb 7oz) or has reached her actual due date (although she'll probably be required to gain more weight than that to be let home). She must show that she can feed well, taking in either breast milk or formula, and she must have gained, and still be gaining, weight. Most babies stay in the special care baby unit for two to three weeks, unless there are serious health problems that need to be dealt with.

Although premature babies may hit milestones slightly later than other babies of the same age, they will generally catch up with their peers by the time they reach two. If you have a premature baby, it is best to look at her development in terms of her estimated rather than actual due date. For example, most babies smile around six weeks while premature babies may smile a little later.

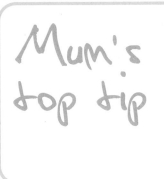

Mum's top tip

My tip is trust your body and if you feel you need pain relief, gently insist until you get it. My daughter was born ten weeks early, weighing 3lb 12oz. My waters broke on a Tuesday morning and I didn't give birth till 1.57am on Friday. Labour itself wasn't too bad, although my contractions hurt a lot. The midwives looking after me didn't actually believe that I was going into labour, so I didn't get gas and air until I started pushing.

Breech birth

A breech baby sits upright in the womb rather than head first. About one baby in four is breech at 28 weeks, although most turn around by 36 weeks. Babies who come early tend to be breech because they haven't turned yet.

Although plenty of women give birth successfully to breech babies, they do pose more of a problem during vaginal delivery. Your baby continues getting his oxygen through the umbilical cord until his head emerges and he can breathe properly. If he comes out bottom first the cord can become squashed and his oxygen supply may be reduced, putting him in danger.

If your pelvis is roomy, and your doctor thinks there is plenty of space for a breech delivery, there is no reason why you shouldn't give birth naturally. If there is insufficient space, or the danger of complications arising, your doctor may advise you to have a Caesarean section (see pages 130–2).

If you go into labour before term (37 weeks) and your baby is breech, you will probably be advised to have a Caesarean because of the risk to your baby's health if you give birth naturally. If you

Mum's top tip

My first baby was breech and I ended up having a Caesarean because he hadn't turned! I healed very quickly. I am 34 weeks pregnant now and this baby is breech too (must run in the family as my mum was a breech baby). One midwife told me to put a bag of frozen peas on my belly and the baby would move away from the cold and turn around. I tried this but all I got was a freezing-cold tummy!

have any concerns, or are unhappy about having a Caesarean, it's best to discuss these issues with the midwives and doctors who are looking after you.

With a breech delivery you are probably more likely to have an episiotomy (see pages 188–91), so that your baby has plenty of room to emerge. Evidence suggests that giving birth in the 'all fours' position can help give your breech baby more room.

Every pregnancy and every woman is different, of course, and you and your baby will be assessed individually to see whether it is safe for you to deliver vaginally.

Can my baby be turned before birth?

Breech babies can be turned using a technique known as external cephalic version (ECV). The Royal College of Obstetricians recommends that ECVs are performed on women expecting a breech baby provided they have reached 37 weeks and have had an uncomplicated pregnancy up until that point.

The ECV must be performed at a hospital because the procedure needs to be carried out by a skilled professional and because of the risk of your baby becoming distressed. You won't need a general anaesthetic but you will need to be monitored because of the risks to your unborn child. You will be given an injection to relax the muscles in your womb and a doctor or midwife will externally turn your baby to face head down. This can be painful for you, but probably not as painful as having a Caesarean section. Talk this procedure through with your midwife if you are worried and ask what your options are if you don't have an ECV.

Never try to turn your baby yourself: this procedure can be dangerous for your baby and must be performed by a skilled medical professional.

Inducing labour

It can be pretty disappointing when your due date comes and goes, and there is no sign of the baby. Most women are offered an induction at roughly 7–14 days past their due date, but each woman will be individually monitored and reviewed.

Generally speaking, the hospital will consider an induction if you reach 42 weeks of pregnancy and there is no evidence that labour has started. This is because there can be increased complications when a pregnancy has gone beyond 42 weeks. In an attempt to prevent problems, the medical staff will induce – which means artificially start labour – at this time.

Some women will be offered an induction before their due date if they are suffering from pre-eclampsia (see pages 102–3) or their waters have been broken for a while but labour has not started.

Typical methods of induction

MEMBRANE SWEEP

A membrane sweep can be a useful way of starting labour before other methods of induction are considered. The midwife gently inserts her finger into the neck of your womb and sweeps around the membranes at the edge of the cervix. This releases substances known as prostaglandins (see opposite) which can kick-start labour. This procedure may be uncomfortable as the cervix can be difficult to reach, and you may feel some irregular contractions immediately afterwards. If the sweep is successful, labour will start within 48 hours.

SYNTHETIC PROSTAGLANDIN

Your body naturally produces prostaglandins, which stimulate the uterus into contracting, but some women may need synthetic prostaglandin to help get labour started. This can be administered by inserting a pessary or gel into the vagina to soften the cervix. You may need more than one dose of prostaglandin to start contractions, with doses being given every six to eight hours.

There are disadvantages to being induced in this way. Once contractions start, you will probably have to be monitored using a foetal heart rate monitor for a while, although once it is established that your labour is going well, you may be taken off the monitor, which will mean you can move around freely again. Most doses of prostaglandin have to be administered in hospital, which can be frustrating if you planned to stay at home for a while until your labour was well under way. Despite much hearsay suggesting that labour induced with synthetic prostaglandin is more painful than labour that begins naturally, there is no actual evidence to support this.

ARTIFICIAL RUPTURE OF THE MEMBRANES

In about one in 20 pregnancies, a woman's waters will break before she goes into labour, and for nine out of ten women labour will start within 24 hours. If your waters have not broken, one way of speeding up contractions is for your doctor to artificially break the bag of membranes surrounding your baby. Once the bag has broken, the amniotic fluid leaks out and the amount of prostaglandins increase, speeding up labour. The procedure is done using a long plastic instrument with a hook at one end. It's not painful; just a little uncomfortable.

SYNTOCINON

Syntocinon is a synthetic hormone that makes the uterus contract, and can be used once the cervix has softened. It is usually administered using an IV (intravenous line), so you won't be able to move around much. You may have be attached to a foetal monitor, as syntocinon can overstimulate the uterus and result in your baby becoming distressed. If this is the case, your midwife will reduce the dose and may give you another drug to slow contractions down.

You will have to be in hospital throughout your induction and early labour, which can be a disappointment if you planned to stay at home for as long as possible during labour.

If you have already been given synthetic prostaglandin, you will not be given syntocinon for at least six hours. Women who are given syntocinon are more likely to need an epidural for the pain as the drug can bring labour on fairly quickly, with relatively little build-up.

Why might I need to be induced?

- If you are 7–14 days over your due date, it is better for your baby to be outside the womb because of the risk of infections she may now be prone to in the uterus.

- If you develop pre-eclampsia (see pages 102–3), the only cure may be delivering your baby.

- If your placenta stops functioning properly, it may be better for your baby to be born and looked after by a medical team.

- If your waters break but contractions do not start, inducing labour is advised as your womb is now open to infection.

- If you have previously had a full-term stillborn baby, early induction may be advised.

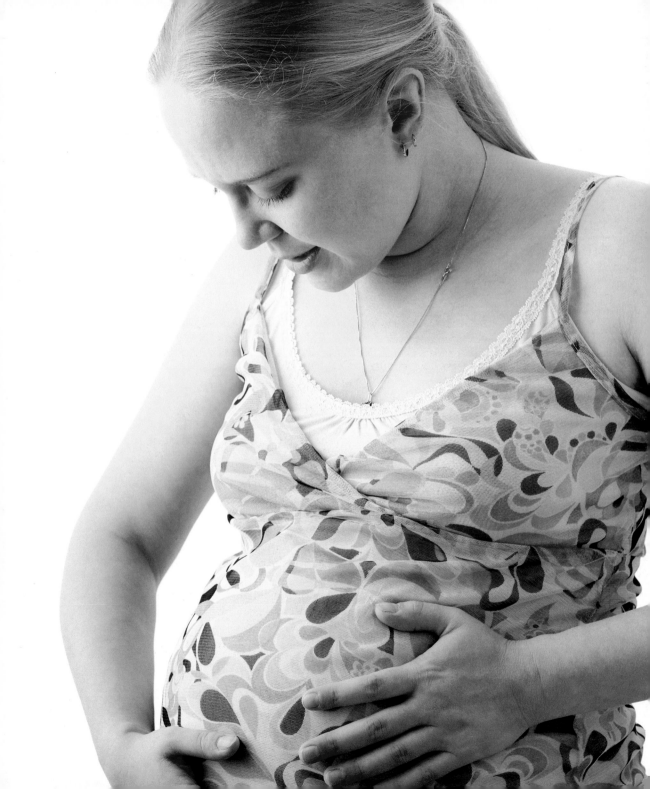

Breathing techniques

Controlled breathing helps you to avoid tensing up while you are having a contraction, making it less painful. It also sends oxygen around your bloodstream and to your baby, which enables your muscles to function more efficiently. Breathing properly helps you ease the tension and distracts you from the pain of labour by giving you something to focus on.

Breathing techniques to help you through labour

AT THE START, FINISH AND BETWEEN CONTRACTIONS

All contractions should start with a cleansing breath. Relax. Breathe in through your nose and out through your mouth. Breathe in and out again, but this time when you breathe out, try to expel all the air in your lungs so your 'out' breath is long and your lungs are empty. It's best to keep this going between contractions in order to establish rhythmical breathing, which will help you to feel calm and in control.

AS YOU FEEL A CONTRACTION COMING

Keep breathing in through your nose and out through your mouth, but speed up your breathing a little. Try not to empty your lungs completely before taking another breath. It may help to make the noise 'hee' on the out breath. When you feel the contraction ending, try to slow down your breath again, expelling all the air from your lungs as you exhale.

WHEN CONTRACTIONS ARE INTENSE
Breathe in quickly and blow out, so your breathing is shallower. It might help to say 'hoo' on the out breath.

IF YOU NEED TO AVOID PUSHING
If your cervix has not fully dilated but you feel the urge to push, use this technique to help you avoid pushing. Visualize a feather or a candle and pant or blow lightly just enough to keep the feather bouncing in the air, or so the candle stays lit but the flame flickers. This can help to distract you from the urge the push.

AS YOU PUSH YOUR BABY OUT
Breathe in deeply. As you breathe out, push downwards with your abdominal muscles.

 For the **gurgle** video on **Breathing techniques for labour and birth**, go to **gurgle.com** and click on **Videos**

top
tips

Before you go into labour

You may feel as if the birth of your child is turning into a full-scale military operation, what with your bag packed and birth plan printed. But forewarned is forearmed, so here are just a few more ideas to help everything run smoothly both before and after the birth.

Top tips on preparing for labour

PRACTISE YOUR DRIVE TO THE HOSPITAL

You probably drive past the hospital all the time, but time how long it takes during the rush hour and when parents are doing the school run, in case valuable minutes are added to your journey. Check with the hospital where the closest car park is for the maternity unit – you don't want to arrive back at your car with your new baby only to find it's been clamped!

COOK FOR THE FREEZER

When you get home from hospital, all you'll want to think about is your newborn baby. You will probably live on a cloud for a while, tending to your newborn's every need, and the last thing to cross your mind will be preparing dinner. It may be useful for you or your partner to cook a few dishes in advance before your baby arrives and stick them in the freezer. Defrost them as needed after your baby is born, and that way you will get a hot meal every day and you can devote your time to your newborn.

top tips

GET YOUR LABOUR AND DELIVERY KIT READY

With your due date looming, it's a good idea to pack a bag with everything you'll need for hospital. Have this ready a few weeks in advance just in case your baby arrives early. (See overleaf for advice on what to pack.)

DON'T FORGET NAPPIES

Don't forget to buy a stock of newborn nappies for when you get home from the hospital. Newborn babies can sometimes get through 8–10 a day and you don't want to run out mid-poo! You will also need sanitary towels for after the birth – buying your own is definitely preferable to the ones the maternity ward give you, which are like cardboard!

SORT OUT CHILDCARE IN ADVANCE

You may go into labour at any time, even at 2 or 3am, so make sure you think about who can look after any other children you have if you and your partner need to make a mad dash to hospital. If they are old enough to understand, explain to them that you have to go away for a few days but you will be back very soon and you love them very much.

DECIDE WHO'S ALLOWED IN THE DELIVERY ROOM...

Make sure your partner or birth partner is briefed about exactly what YOU want during labour, birth and afterwards. This might mean requesting that no one, not even your mum, comes to see you while in labour. If your family is insisting on hanging around until the baby is born, you can always ask a midwife to have a word with them if it is stressing you out. Even though you can have who you like with you in the delivery room, the midwife can always tell family members that the hospital has a one-visitor policy (which might be useful when your mother-in-law turns up unannounced!).

...AND KEEP VISITORS AT BAY

After you have had your baby, you may also be bombarded with masses of visitors, so make sure you have a word with your partner or midwife if you feel they are swamping your bedside and are too much to cope with. If you are trying to establish breastfeeding or you feel sleep deprived, you may want to send any visitors away. Tell them to come and see you when you are at home and will appreciate the help!

top
tips

Your labour bag: what to pack

It's important to pack the right items in your labour bag because you don't want to have to send your family and friends out buying pyjamas for you or clothes for your baby. Below are gurgle's suggestions for what you'll need during your hospital stay.

FOR WHEN YOU'RE IN LABOUR:
- Your maternity notes
- Birth plan
- Loose clothing for giving birth in, such as an old nightshirt or big T-shirt. Pack a few in case they get messy
- Warm socks and slippers
- Toothbrush, toothpaste, mouthwash and your make-up bag
- Hairbrush and hair bands (Alice bands are great for keeping your hair back during labour)
- A pillow if you want your own
- Deodorant and lip balm
- Essential oils if you've chosen to use them
- Massage oil or lotion if you'd like to be massaged during labour
- TENS machine, if you're planning to use one
- Mobile phone and a list of numbers for your midwife, doula, friends and relatives
- Non-perishable snacks and drinks for you and your partner
- Books, magazines – anything to keep you occupied in the early stages of labour
- CD or MP3 player
- If it's hot, you may need a mini fan or a face spray.

FOR AFTER THE BIRTH:
- One or two nightdresses, preferably 100% cotton, in a loose style with a button-down front for breastfeeding
- Dressing gown and slippers
- **Very important:** shower gel, moisturizer, shampoo and conditioner. Treat yourself to some luxurious brands – you deserve to feel pampered after giving birth!
- Maternity sanitary towels and knickers
- If you plan to breastfeed: nursing bra, breast pads and nipple cream/guards. Breast pump (this is optional as most maternity units have breast pumps, but as they are usually shared between women, you might want to use your own – check with your maternity unit)
- Shawl or pashmina, so you can look glamorous when visitors arrive (optional).

FOR YOUR BABY:
- Two/three newborn Babygros (sleepsuits)
- Two bodysuits (with sleeves if it's cold, sleeveless if it's warm)
- One pair of socks or booties
- Baby blanket (cellular blanket)
- Baby hat and scratch mittens
- A going-home outfit. If it is winter, make sure you pack a warm cardigan; in the summer you'll need a hat to keep the sun off your baby's eyes
- One pack of newborn-size nappies
- Cotton wool or baby wipes
- One pack of muslin cloths – essential for pretty much everything, but mainly for mopping up when your baby brings up milk.

Essential items

At no other time in your life are you faced with such a mindboggling array of things to buy as when you are expecting a baby. And if it's not difficult enough sorting out the essential purchases from the things you can live without, once you've decided what you need there are countless different brands, styles and features to choose from. But fear not – read on for all you need to help you make all the right purchases for you and your baby.

Choosing a car seat

It's essential that you have a car seat ready for your baby by the time you give birth – if you are giving birth in a hospital you won't be allowed to leave without one.

The type of car seat you need depends on your child's weight and height. Babies should always be placed in rearward-facing baby seats and should not be moved to a forward-facing seat until they weigh at least 9kgs.

When deciding whether to buy a particular car seat, if it is not clear, contact the manufacturer of the seat first to check if it will fit your car. If so, you can always ask to try it out in your car and make sure you're comfortable using it before you buy it. And always check that the seat meets United Nations standard Regulation 44.03 or 44.04 - look for the 'E' mark.

Pushchairs and prams: things to think about

New prams and pushchairs are not cheap, so it's important to get the right one for you. To help narrow things down keep in mind two important questions: will it fit your needs and will it fit your baby's needs?

THREE-IN-ONE PRAM AND PUSHCHAIR COMBINATION

Suitable for newborn to toddler, these offer a padded carrycot which fits into the 'chassis', the pram's frame, and a separate pushchair unit which locks into the chassis.

TWO-IN-ONE PRAM AND PUSHCHAIR COMBINATION

As above, but the carrycot and pushchair are the same unit. With the seat fully reclined, it can be used as a pram for the first few months. As the baby gets older, the seat can be converted to create a pushchair.

Pros ● The seat unit can usually be positioned to face towards or away from you ● Generally has a larger-wheeled chassis which means better suspension.

Cons ● Expensive ● Can be cumbersome ● The large wheels make manoeuvring more tricky.

THREE-WHEELER PUSHCHAIRS

With their robust design and gripping threaded tyres, three-wheelers are great for all sorts of terrain and/or jogging as well as everyday use. They must have a fully reclinable seat if they are to be used for a newborn.

Pros ● Can be taken places it would be impossible to take a regular pram, eg: muddy fields ● May come with a storage bag for easy transportation ● Fold flat for easy storage.

Cons ● Can be heavy to lift ● Can be expensive ● Quite cumbersome if being used in town ● You will need to pump up the tyres fairly regularly.

TRAVEL SYSTEMS – FROM CAR SEAT TO PUSHCHAIR

These include either a carrycot, pushchair and car seat, or a pushchair and car seat. The various components attach to the chassis. It might seem expensive buying the three things together but it can actually be cheaper to buy them as a package. Make sure that the car seat is compatible with the make of your car.

Pros ● Convenience: you buy a carrycot, pushchair and car seat in one go ● A baby can be moved from pram to car or vice versa without being woken.

Cons ● The car seat is generally only for babies up to 13kg/29lbs (approximately 9–12 months), so you will have to invest in another one fairly soon.

BASIC BUGGIES AND PUSHCHAIRS

These are lightweight, versatile and simple to use, and most can be used from birth (they need to recline fully as newborns need to lie completely flat). Depending on what you pay, extras may include adjustable handles, a sun/rain canopy and shopping basket. Do make sure that the pushchair you choose is sturdy, comfortable and well-padded and that it is also rain- and wind-proof.

Pros ● Less expensive than travel systems etc ● Lightweight frame ● Compact when folded ● A number of lie-back positions.

Cons ● Your baby generally lies facing away from you ● Not as comfortable for sleeping in as a pram unit which comes with a carrycot and mattress.

DOUBLE BUGGIES

If you are expecting twins, or you have a baby as well as a child who still uses a pushchair, you may want to think about buying a double buggy. There are two types: side-by-side buggies (where the seats are next to each other) and tandem buggies (where one seat is behind the other). Many people with children close in age find side-by-side buggies best; with tandem buggies only the backseat reclines fully, and a newborn needs to lie flat.

Be prepared for a shock when you first try out a double buggy: they are much heavier and more cumbersome than single buggies. But with a bit off practice you'll be flying down the streets like Lewis Hamilton.

SIDE-BY-SIDE BUGGIES

Pros ● Almost all allow you to recline each seat separately, so one child can sleep if the other wants to sit up.

Cons ● Although all are designed to fit through the standard UK door width of 79cms, with some side-by-side buggies it's a tighter squeeze than others.

TANDEM BUGGIES

Pros ● Easier than the side-by-side buggy to get through doorways.

Cons ● Might be too big for some small spaces, eg, lifts ● The folding mechanism can be quite tricky ● Bulky when folded.

Baby carriers and slings

Make sure you try on any carrier you are thinking of buying, with your baby inside it, or, if you want to try on a few, a good shop should have sandbags you can use to emulate your baby rather than having to keep moving him in and out of them.

FRONT CARRIERS

Front carriers are usually quite simple in design and easy to use. Most are suitable from birth, and those that are will generally have a smaller insert in which a newborn can be placed so that he doesn't get lost in the carrier. Your baby is comfortably supported by his bottom and/or crotch. Front carriers usually have a padded headrest – but always ensure the headrest is folded down if you are carrying your baby away from you so that it does not pose a suffocation risk.

Pros ● Lightweight ● Easy to use ● Can be put on and taken off without waking a sleeping baby.

Cons ● Are only really suitable for small babies ● Needs to be taken off to breastfeed ● Can strain the shoulders if worn for long periods of time, so make sure the carrier has well padded shoulder straps.

BACKPACK CARRIERS

Backpacks are usually designed for babies six months and older who can hold their heads up, up to babies around 18kg (40lb). They generally have metal frames, padded shoulder straps and a cushioned head-rest and crotch seat. Some will have a storage pockets and a detachable sunshade too.

Pros ● Versatile, comfortable, stable ● Great for long walks and hiking ● Allows your baby to see more of the world around him

Cons ● Can be difficult to put your baby into ● Do not generally support the head and neck so only suitable for older babies ● Difficult for a baby to fall asleep in ● The whole carrier must be taken off to comfort or breastfeed a baby ● Can be pricey.

SLINGS

Slings are a wide swathe of cloth supported by a single shoulder strap. They can be padded or unpadded and may or may not have rings, which are used to adjust and secure the material. They are generally suitable for children up to 9kg (20lb).

Pros ● No fiddling with buckles and straps ● Not bulky ● Some have a breastfeeding position ● Can be used in a variety of positions ● The baby can be put into a car seat in the sling and just lifted out again – no more heavy car seat to carry ● Machine washable

Cons ● Many do not have safety restraints ● The straps can be too short for those of a larger build ● Many slings have very deep sides, meaning the baby is unable to see out ● Despite manufacturers' guidelines to the contrary, many users say they find slings unsuitable for babies over 4.5–6.8kg (10–15lb)

LONG TIED WRAPS
These are strips of cloth typically 12 foot long which are wrapped around the parent's and the baby's bodies and then secured by a knot. They can be wrapped in various ways so that the baby is facing forwards or back and located on either the parent's chest or back.

Pros ● Extremely versatile – baby can be carried in many different ways ● Flexible for breastfeeding ● Lightweight and soft for parent and baby ● Machine washable

Cons ● Wrapping can be tricky to begin with ● Not able to put it on quickly ● Some babies find it too restrictive ● Doesn't offer much in the way of padding so can become uncomfortable

Changing tables

Another one of the items of equipment you'll use most when you have a new baby is a changing station as, you guessed, babies get through a lot of nappies in a day!

A changing table (sometimes called a changing station) is a specially designed unit which will help you keep all your nappy-changing essentials – wipes, nappy bags etc – organized in one place. It's not an essential purchase by any means but it can make your life a whole lot easier. Look for a changing table that is stable and firm with an easy-to-clean surface. It's also advisable to choose one with raised sides to guard your baby from falling (although you should never leave a baby unattended on a changing table or any raised surface).

Pros • All equipment is in one area • Compact • If you are recovering from the birth, using one puts far less strain on your back and any stitches.

Cons • There is a risk that your baby might fall, which increases as your baby becomes more mobile • They are bulky and cannot be used when travelling.

Beds

We all hope we're going to be blessed with a good sleeper, and hopefully the following information will help to ensure your baby is! Here's gurgle's lowdown on everything you will need for your new baby – and you – to get a safe (and preferably long) night's sleep.

MOSES BASKETS AND CARRYCOTS

Moses baskets are small, light, portable cots. They usually come with their own fabric-covered foam mattress. They have handles, and so are easily transportable and can be carried wherever you go, be it the living room or a restaurant.

Carrycots are an alternative to Moses baskets. If you have a three-in-one pram, you will already have a carrycot as part of it, but stand-alone carrycots are also available. These will usually come with a chassis, which resembles a pram and folds flat.

Pros • They're portable • Take up little space • You may already have a carrycot as part of your pram.

Cons • They don't last for long – most Moses baskets and carrycots are only suitable for babies up to around three months, although of course it depends on the size of the individual baby.

CRIBS

Another option for the first few months of your baby's life is a crib. A crib is larger than a Moses basket and will therefore last your baby a bit longer; hopefully up until the age of six months (again this is dependent on the size of your baby). A crib should not be used once your baby can sit up or pull herself up. Cribs are generally made from wood and have a gliding or rocking action designed to help your baby fall to sleep.

Pros • Rocking motion to help your baby fall asleep • Last longer than a Moses basket.

Cons • Your baby will grow out of it by six months.

COTS

Cots come in an array different shapes and sizes. Before you buy a cot, check that is carries the British Standards Institution (BSI) number BS EN 716:1996, indicating that it complies with current safety standards.

When choosing a cot, you need to think about how long you want your baby to sleep in it: if you are hoping that your baby will spend the first few years of his life in the cot, then the bigger the better. However, if you are planning to move your baby into a bed by the age of two or three, then it's best to buy a fairly small cot with a view to buying a single bed later on.

Pros • Larger than Moses basket/carrycot/crib • Your baby has more room to move • One cot can be used for twins • Last a couple of years.

Cons • Not portable • Expensive.

Happy birth day

Am I in labour?

Weeks before your baby is due, you'll probably start to notice signs that your body is getting ready for labour.

ENGAGEMENT

Engagement is one of the physical signs that labour is imminent. In order for your baby's journey through the birth canal to begin, he will move himself deeper into your pelvis. In most cases, he will be head down – the optimum position for delivery. If this is your first pregnancy, the baby will move down roughly 2–3 weeks before labour starts, but with subsequent pregnancies, your uterine muscles will have stretched so that your baby doesn't have to move so far down.

NESTING INSTINCT

A nesting instinct is shown by pregnant women in the form of an uncontrollable urge to clean their house and everything around them. Females in the animal kingdom exhibit the same behaviour just before their offspring arrive. You may want to

Mum's top tip

I found that going for walks helped me go into labour. Other suggestions are to eat a hot curry, have sex, or make some raspberry leaf tea. Once labour had started, I got relief from standing up and rocking gently to and fro, from foot to foot. I let gravity take over and help my baby's way into the world! When my contractions started, they felt like period pains so I asked my partner to rub my back and my bump (very gently) and I found that really soothing!

clean everything you see, or throw out anything old and grubby, or you may retreat into familiar company and the comfort of your own home. The nesting instinct can appear around the fifth month, but if you are close to 40 weeks pregnant, it may indicate the onset of labour.

BRAXTON HICKS CONTRACTIONS

Braxton Hicks contractions, named after the man who first identified them, are a sign of your uterus practising for the stronger contractions of labour. They are much weaker, of course, and normally painless. They can be uncomfortable, however, and sometimes quite intense. They start with a tightening feeling in your uterus and spread downwards before relaxing. They typically last 15–20 seconds but sometimes can go on for much longer. If you find them painful, keeping active can help or changing position (see pages 176–77), or you may prefer to lie down when you are having them.

A SHOW

A show is one of the more obvious signs that labour is on its way. A plug of mucus seals your cervix and protects it from infection. If your cervix dilates enough, the mucus plug may become dislodged, and will appear as a sticky, brown/pink substance. Even though labour itself may be hours or even days away, you must inform the hospital if you have a show because once the mucus plug is gone from the opening of the cervix, the baby is vulnerable to infection.

VAGINAL DISCHARGE

Some women notice increased vaginal discharge as their cervix softens. It may look like egg white, but can also have a pinkish appearance.

MEMBRANE RUPTURE (WATERS BREAKING)

Membrane rupture, or waters breaking, is when the amniotic sac that contains your baby breaks at the end of pregnancy and the amniotic fluid leaks out. Most women go into labour 24 hours after their waters break, because the rupture signals the release of prostaglandins, which stimulate contractions. Once your waters break, be careful not to put anything into your vagina and have showers rather than baths as infections can now get to your baby. Once your waters have broken, call your midwife or maternity unit to let them know. They will probably ask how much fluid leaked out and what the consistency was like, so make a note of this. They will advise you whether to wait at home, or come into the hospital.

REGULAR CONTRACTIONS

When your irregular contractions are replaced by more consistent ones, which get stronger, come every five minutes and last roughly 45-60 seconds, you are in established labour and should phone the hospital or your midwife. You are not in established labour if your contractions are irregular (sometimes occurring every three minutes, sometimes every 5-10 minutes), or if they don't intensify over time but lessen if you walk about or lie down. The rule of thumb seems to be, if you can't speak during a contraction you are in labour proper and should phone your hospital.

Most women can tell when they are in established labour. But if you are still in doubt, phone your midwife who can help put your mind at rest, telling you to rest at home, or will ask you to come into the maternity unit to be examined.

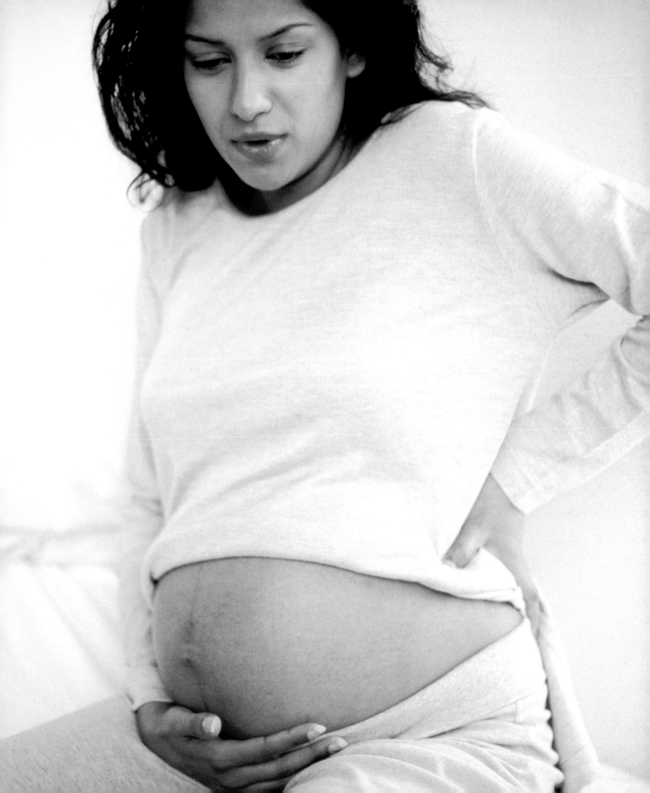

When should I go to hospital?

It may be tempting to rush to hospital as soon as you feel the first twinge of a contraction, but the longer you stay at home, the better. The last thing you want is to be waiting around for hours at the hospital, where the atmosphere is unfamiliar and could make you tense, when you could be enjoying the comforts of your own home. Similarly, you don't want to arrive at the hospital only to be told you have to go home again.

Staying at home during early labour has many advantages, such as your bed and bathroom being nearby (in some maternity wards the delivery room may not have a bathroom attached).

Equipment for early labour

BIRTHING BALL

You may have seen these huge inflatable balls at the hospital but you can buy or hire one for home. Lots of women find a birthing ball gives comfort: you can lie on it, sit and rock on it or lean over it for support. Many women also report using them after their baby is born to sit on and rock their baby to sleep.

TENS MACHINE

A TENS machine (see page 119) is a popular, non-invasive form of pain relief that works by blocking the pain signals from reaching your brain, so that you feel less pain. If you do hire or buy a machine, it is a good idea to practise with it first before you go into labour, as it's a device that can be tricky to get the hang of, but very effective once you do. (For more options for non-invasive pain relief, see pages 178–9.)

When to leap into action

If your waters break, or your contractions are five minutes apart and get stronger over time, or if you experience any vaginal bleeding, it is time to head to the hospital. Phone your midwife to explain which stage of labour you think you are at, and she will talk through the details and advise you what to do next. Even if you go to hospital at this stage, you may still be told to go home and return only when contractions become unbearable.

Hospital admission

When you arrive at the hospital, you may be shown to your own room, or to a special room for women who have just been admitted. Your midwife will ask a series of questions about your labour so far. It is important that you bring your maternity notes with you as they contain all the information about your pregnancy. Typical questions may include: Have your waters broken? Have you experienced any contractions; if so how long and how far apart? When did you last eat? Have you had a show, or any vaginal bleeding? In addition:

- Your blood pressure will be checked, along with your pulse, breathing and temperature, and you may be asked to provide a urine sample
- You will have an internal examination to see if your cervix has dilated at all. If it hasn't, you may be sent home until you are in active labour
- Your midwife will feel your tummy to check where the baby is lying and what position she is lying in
- You might show your birth plan (if you have one) to your midwife and discuss your preferences for the birth

What can or can't I do in early labour?

If you can manage to stay at home during early labour, you will probably be thankful later – the longer you can stay in your own, relaxed environment, the better. You might think that you won't be able to do anything once you go into labour, but it depends on how fast things are moving. It can be a long while before things get going properly.

Can I eat or drink?

You can certainly eat and drink as normal in early labour, and it might be a good idea to do so as you will need all your energy for the delivery itself. Don't worry if you don't feel like eating – lots of women actually feel sick during labour and won't want to eat at all.

WHAT TO EAT

If you are hungry, eat little and often, so as not to burden your stomach, and nothing too rich and spicy. It's best to stick to the following sorts of food:

- Toast
- Bananas
- Raisins
- Pasta
- Cereals
- Rice cakes
- Rice

WHAT TO DRINK

Drink plenty of water throughout your labour so that you do not get dehydrated. Water will also increase the number of times you need to wee, which will help you keep mobile during labour. Some health professionals swear by sports energy drinks while others don't recommend them – ask your midwife for her opinion. Tea and coffee are not recommended, because of the caffeine content, but fruit juices such as apple juice can be refreshing and hydrating.

What if I need an anaesthetic and I have just eaten?

If you need a general anaesthetic and have eaten prior to the operation there is a small risk that the food in your stomach could be regurgitated and inhaled through the lungs. However, as you fall asleep the nurse will apply a little pressure to the cricoid cartilage in your neck to close the junction between the gullet and the lungs, and this will stop any food from reaching the lungs.

More often than not, Caesarean sections are performed under an epidural or spinal blocks these days (see pages 130–1), which pose no risk as far as eating during labour is concerned.

How can I spend my time?

Some women go to see a film with their partner in early labour, or even go out for dinner. Most women just want to relax and prepare themselves for the birth. Now can be a good time to look through your labour bag to make sure you have everything you need. (For what to pack in your bag, see pages 148–9.)

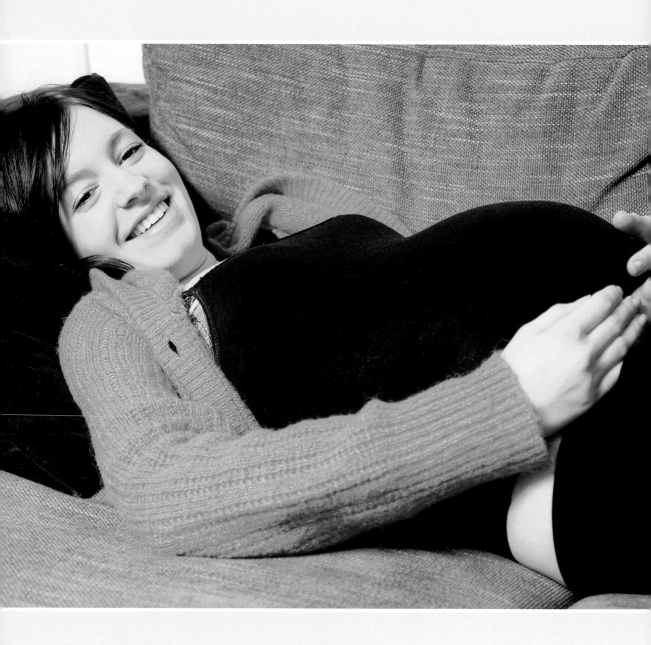

Happy birth day

How can I relax?

Taking a warm bath (unless your waters have broken as this can increase the chances of infection), going for a gentle walk or practising your breathing exercises are all excellent preparation for labour. The important thing is to try and unwind. You are bound to feel a little nervous, but trust in yourself and your body, and then you will be able to relax and go with the flow.

Keep well hydrated and follow your physical cues. If you feel like walking around, walk around; if you feel like lying down, then do so. Avoid strenuous activity or anything that is likely to make you feel stressed. And avoid having sex if your waters have broken, you have had a show, or you have any vaginal bleeding.

If you have other children, it might be a good idea to get a babysitter to look after them, so that you are not worrying about them. If you have arranged for them to stay with a friend or relative, now may be the time to take them there or have them picked up.

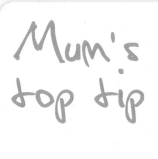

My heartfelt advice is to try to relax and not worry about what your labour will be like. Your body already knows what to do and the medical staff are there to do the rest. Speak to your birth partner before you go into labour, discuss your birth plan with him or her, and let him know what you do and don't want. Do your research so you can make the right choices for you, and don't be bullied into anything! It is your right to choose where and how you have your baby.

What are the stages of labour?

While every woman has a different experience of childbirth, she will still go through the three stages of labour, unless she has an elective Caesarean before labour begins. It can be helpful to view your labour in these stages, so that once you reach the end of one stage, you will know you are that much closer to meeting your baby.

Your cervix lies at the top of your vagina, and must fully dilate in order for your baby to come out. In the first stage, your uterus will tense and relax and cause a contraction. Contractions get more intense with fewer gaps in between as labour progresses. When the cervix widens and thins enough for the baby to pass through, the second stage begins and your baby in born. The third stage is the delivery of the placenta, your baby's life support system in your womb. These make up the three stages of labour.

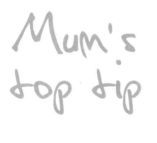

Mum's top tip

Don't worry unduly – not all labours are long and painful and when the baby is in your arms you'll forget all you've been through. When my due date arrived, I waited all day and at 12.15am I felt my first contraction. At 1am I went to the toilet and had a sudden urge to push. I called my midwife, who took one look at me and told me to push!!! By 2am, I had my baby boy in my arms. It wasn't the birth I had planned but it was the best experience I've ever had!!

Stage 1

Stage 1 begins with the onset of regular contractions and lasts until the cervix has softened, thinned and dilated (opened) to 10cm (4in). Even though this stage is the longest, don't be disheartened. One misconception about labour is that you spend hours and hours in pain, but between contractions, especially in the first stages of labour, you will probably be able to read a magazine, eat some lunch or chat happily to your birth partner. There will also be time to rest and gather your strength for the second stage of labour, which is a bit more challenging. It is easier to see stage 1 further divided into three sections:

THE LATENT STAGE

Many women will have regular contractions as the cervix dilates, and these can vary from mild – so mild that they hardly distract you – to strong and painful. Some women may not even know that they are in labour during these very early contractions, and could become several centimetres dilated before they realize it. Most women describe early labour pains as being like heavy menstrual cramps that get stronger and more intense as labour progresses. It's important to note the length and strength of your actual contractions, rather than the time between them. If they last 30–40 seconds and you are able to enjoy a cup of tea in between, you are unlikely to be in established labour.

Women are generally advised to stay at home during the early part of labour, until their contractions get stronger and more regular, coming every five minutes and lasting 45–60 seconds. This is when you are in established labour, also known as the active stage.

THE ACTIVE STAGE

This stage is shorter and lasts about three to five hours on average. You are in active labour when your cervix has dilated to 3–4cm (1¼–1½in). Contractions become longer, with a shorter gap in between. It may be at this stage that you decide you would be more comfortable at the hospital than at home (unless you are planning a home birth – see pages 118–21). The contractions can be painful, and it is at this point that you may require pain relief. By the end of this stage, your cervix will be either fully dilated or almost fully dilated. (For options on pain relief in labour, see pages 178–83.)

TRANSITIONAL STAGE

The transitional stage acts as a bridge between stages 1 and 2. You will be fully dilated, or nearly so, and about to enter the 'pushing' stage. For some women the transitional stage is a period of rest – the contractions can ease while your body prepares for your baby to come out. For others, this stage makes them behave irrationally, and they can lose heart. With encouragement such feelings will pass, however, and you will soon be moving on to the next stage. Your midwife will recognize that you are in the transitional stage, and will probably tell you how close you are to meeting your baby. You may feel a very strong urge to bear down or push, but if your cervix hasn't fully dilated, you will be encouraged to breathe through the contractions and wait until your cervix has completely opened.

 For the **gurgle** video on **Breathing techniques for labour and birth**, go to **gurgle.com** and click on **Videos**

Stage 2

Stage 2 begins when you are fully dilated and ends with the birth of your baby. The contractions you now feel are different from those experienced in stage 1, giving you an overwhelming desire to bear down and push out your baby. If you push when your cervix has not dilated fully, it will swell and take longer to open. This is why your midwife will only allow you to push once you are fully dilated. If you breathe slowly through each contraction and use gas and air, it can help to open up the cervix. (For more on breathing techniques in labour, see pages 144–5.)

At this stage, most women do not need to be guided, and they will go with what their body is telling them to do. Some women worry about the sounds they make during the delivery of their baby, but if grunting, groaning (or screaming at your partner) helps you to deal with each contraction, it will help make the birth easier, and you should go with it.

PUSHING

If you can, try to keep your pushing smooth, and make your muscular effort slow and steady to avoid putting pressure on the perineum (the area between the anus and vagina). Try not to hold your breath when you're pushing, and push for as long as you are able. Most women prefer to be in a more upright position at this stage as gravity helps the baby move downwards and you don't have to do as much work. It is also helpful to relax your pelvic floor and anal muscles as much as possible as you are pushing. This may make you urinate or pass a stool, but this is nothing to be embarrassed about. It happens to lots of women and your midwife will have seen it plenty of times before. This stage may only take five or ten minutes for women who have already had a baby; for first-time mums it usually takes about an hour, although it can take much longer.

CROWNING

When your baby is about to be born, your anal area and perineum will bulge as your baby's head becomes visible at your vaginal opening, and you will probably feel a stinging sensation. This is called crowning. Your baby's head may slip back up the birth canal a little between contractions, but with each one he will move a little further forwards again. It can take a couple of contractions after it has crowned for the head to emerge, usually pointing downwards, and your baby will twist so that his shoulders are in a better position to come out. Your midwife may ask you to stop pushing and pant at this stage, to reduce the risk of tearing if the baby is delivered too quickly. The rest of his body should slip out easily once his head and shoulders are through, although some women may need forceps or a ventouse to help them (see pages 186–7). An episiotomy (see pages 188–91) may also be necessary to widen the vaginal opening to enable your baby to come out.

ONCE YOUR BABY IS BORN

Your baby will be covered in blood and vernix, the substance which protected his skin while he was inside you. He will be wrapped in towels to keep him warm, while the mucus is wiped from his nose and mouth and his airways are checked. If everything is as it should be and your baby is doing well, you can relax, cuddle and introduce yourself to him. If you are planning to breastfeed, now is a good time to try with your midwife on hand to help.

Stage 3

Stage 3 is the stage from the birth of your baby to the delivery of the placenta. Some women prefer to wait for the placenta to deliver naturally, which can take slightly longer than if drugs are used. If you put your baby to your breast, it can help to speed things along. This is because breastfeeding your baby stimulates hormones that encourage the placenta to disengage. Blood loss can be a little heavier if you are having a natural stage 3, but this shouldn't be a problem if you have had a straightforward delivery and are in good health.

You can also choose to be injected with a drug called Syntometrine, which contains a synthetic hormone that encourages the uterus to contract and expel the placenta. You will feel a contraction and the midwife will gently tug on the umbilical cord until the placenta comes out. If you had an induction, an epidural or a forceps or ventouse delivery, it may be advised that the third stage is managed with drugs. If you definitely do not want a managed third stage, remember to include this in your birth plan and let your midwife know.

Positions for delivery

The traditional image of a woman in labour shows her lying on her back, but nowadays you are encouraged to remain upright and to keep as active as possible. Many women worry about what they will look like in different positions, but the best approach is to put your embarrassment aside and find a position that feels natural and comfortable for you. Use gravity to help encourage your baby to move down into your pelvis and try to keep as active as possible.

SQUATTING

Squatting encourages your baby to descend quickly and makes pushing easier. Squatting is ideal if you are having a water birth (see pages 122–3) as it can be a tricky position to maintain on dry land, whereas water will support your weight. If you are not in water, your birth partner can help support you.

KNEELING

Kneeling on something soft, and either being supported by your birth partner or resting your hands on your bed, can help to stretch your pelvic ligaments, while a slight rocking movement backwards and forwards may help ease the pain.

STANDING

Standing with support or leaning over a worktop uses gravity to help your baby move downwards.

SITTING UPRIGHT

This can be a great position if you have been standing or squatting and feel tired, or if you have had an epidural and want to remain upright.

top tips

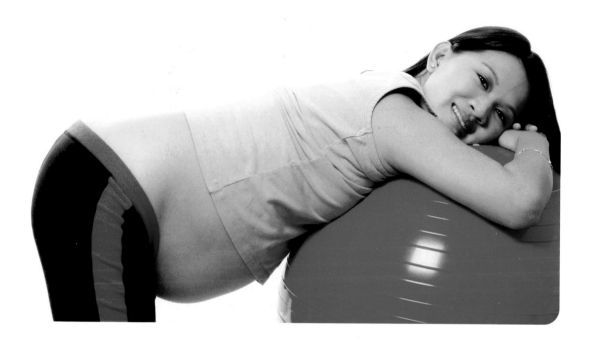

LYING ON YOUR SIDE

This is a useful position if you have had an epidural, or if you want to take the pressure off your cervix. If the baby is coming too quickly, this position can slow things down. Your upper leg should be raised to open your pelvis as much as possible – your birth partner can help support it.

STANDING WITH BENT KNEES

Stand with your birth partner supporting you from behind or in front, letting him or her take your weight. Bend your knees and push against the floor.

top tips

 For the **gurgle** video on **Positions for delivery**,
go to **gurgle.com** and click on **Videos**

Natural pain relief in labour

Most women are perfectly capable of giving birth with little or no pain relief and lots of women opt for a more natural approach. The advantages of this are that you are not introducing any drugs into you or your baby's system, and although you will be able to feel the pain, you can manage it with a variety of methods.

STAYING ACTIVE
Lots of women swear by staying active and keeping on their feet. Most births depicted in films or on television show a women lying on her back. However, staying upright and letting gravity help your baby to descend can make your labour time much faster and contractions easier to deal with. The best option is to go with your instincts. If you feel like walking around, kneeling or rocking, go for it. Alternatively, if you feel like lying down, there is nothing wrong with that either.

TENS MACHINE
TENS machines work by sending small electrical impulses that block the pain of contractions (see page 119). The advantages are that they can be used at home or in the hospital, and they have no effect on your baby. The downside is that they generally have to be hired (although some maternity units do have TENS machines, so make sure you ask beforehand). Please note that TENS machines cannot be used in a birthing pool.

CONTROLLED BREATHING
Breathing properly can help ease the pain of contractions, because it will help you relax and feel in control, enabling you to give birth more easily. Practise taking slow deep breaths and trying not to think about anything except your breathing. It may help to focus your mind if you count up to five when you breathe in and out. (For more on breathing, see pages 144–5.)

RELAXATION

Breathing is part of relaxation, of course, but music can also help. Most maternity units have CD players in their birthing suites, so you can listen to whatever music makes you feel calm and in control.

WATER

Water can play a big part in having a baby, from swimming when you are pregnant to giving birth in a birthing pool (see pages 122–3). A warm bath can ease the pain of contractions and relax your muscles and any tension you are carrying in your body. A hot-water bottle on your back can work in the same way, and might be handy if you are on your way to hospital in a car and experiencing contractions.

MASSAGE

Massage can be a great help, so it may be wise to run through some massage techniques with your birth partner before you go into labour. Kneading your lower back can be effective if you are experiencing backache. Massage can also help your birth partner feel he or she is involved and helping in some way.

HYPNOTHERAPY

Hypnotherapy works by causing the subconscious part of your mind to govern the conscious part. From 34 weeks onwards you can attend courses for self-hypnosis techniques for use in labour, including positive visualization and focusing attention away from the pain. Ask your midwife for recommended pregnancy hypnotherapy courses in your area. (See also the section on HypnoBirthing, pages 124–5.)

NATURAL REMEDIES

Essential oils are a great way to relieve tension and anxiety during labour. Studies have shown that these natural remedies can help relieve the pain of labour and reduce the likelihood of medical intervention. Jasmine, clary sage, rose oil and lavender are just some of the oils that can help. Check beforehand that all the oils you choose are suitable for pregnancy and birth.

What are the medical options?

Even if you plan to have a natural delivery, it is good to bear in mind the medical pain relief available to you, just in case you need other options when labour starts.

Types of pain relief

GAS AND AIR (ENTONOX)

Also known as entonox, gas and air is a mixture of nitrous oxide and oxygen and is inhaled through a mouthpiece or a face mask. You can control how much you have and it helps you to establish a breathing pattern. Gas and air works by numbing the pain centres in the brain and hence dulling the pain of the contraction. You will feel light-headed and floaty, but you will still feel some pain. It is perfectly safe for you and your baby, and you can use it alongside other methods of pain relief. If you are planning a home birth, your midwife can bring gas and air cannisters to your home.

Disadvantages: Gas and air can make some mothers feel slightly nauseous.

Mum's top tip

I would say just go with the flow and if you feel you need an epidural, then ask for it. I had an epidural with both my first two children and it was fantastic! I even slept through labour and they woke me just before it was time to push. However, when I started in labour with my third child, it was very quick and I couldn't have any pain relief - not even gas and air - but it was great. So I've experienced no pain at all and full-on pain!

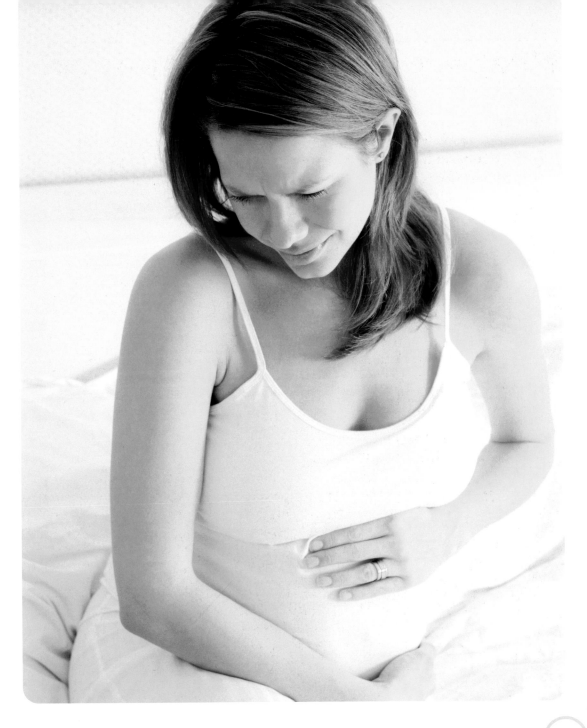

PETHIDINE AND MEPTAZINOL

Pethidine and meptazinol are narcotic drugs which, once injected, induce drowsiness and help to reduce pain. They take roughly 20 minutes to work and can last for three to four hours, when you may need another dose. They work by stimulating receptors in the brain and spinal cord that dull the messages telling your brain you are in pain. The advantages of these drugs are that they are quick to administer – usually just an injection in your bottom or thigh – and are available at most maternity units. They also help to relieve tension and anxiety, so if you feel particularly stressed they might be a good option.

Disadvantages: The drugs can cross through to the placenta which can make your baby drowsy after birth. For this reason, it isn't advisable to have them too close to delivery. You will also become very drowsy and perhaps not able to move about so much, which can in turn slow down labour.

EPIDURAL

The nerves from your spine to your lower back pass through an area called the epidural space. An anaesthetic drug can be injected into this space via a fine tube or catheter. This blocks the nerve messages and causes numbness from your bump downwards – you won't be able to feel any contractions. An epidural can be useful if you are suffering from high blood pressure, as it can bring the pressure down. Having one will not affect your baby in any way.

Disadvantages: An epidural has to be administered by an anaesthetist, who may not always be available at short notice or in the middle of the night. If you are thinking about having an epidural, tell your midwife when you are admitted, or as soon as you decide to have one.

Another downside is that you must keep very still when your back is being injected, which can be tricky if you have a contraction. Movement is totally restricted once the epidural starts to work, and this can slow labour down, so a drip may be needed to speed things up again. For this reason, you may also have a catheter fitted for draining urine, as you won't be able to walk or move around much. You won't feel any contractions so you will probably be told when to push, which can increase the need for a forceps or ventouse delivery (see pages 186–7).

Some women find that an epidural numbs only one side of their body or only a small part of their tummy. There is also a risk of a severe headache if the needle accidentally pierces the sheath around the spinal cord. This can be fixed, once your baby is born, by a procedure which seals the hole made by the epidural needle. Another disadvantage is that you can feel very out of control with an epidural because you have little sensation in your body and cannot feel the contractions, so that the midwife or doctor will need to tell you exactly when to push.

Despite these disadvantages, an epidural is one of the most effective forms of pain relief.

SPINAL BLOCK

A spinal block works in much the same way as an epidural, with the anaesthetic being injected instead into the fluid surrounding the spinal cord. Spinal blocks have become increasingly popular for use in Caesarean sections or emergency obstetric procedures because they work very quickly – almost instantaneously. The spinal block only lasts for an hour or so, so it is not long enough to provide pain relief throughout labour.

Disadvantages: As with an epidural, an anaesthetist is required to administer the drug, so one has to be available. Most women have to have a urinary catheter in place during and after the procedure as movement will be restricted for the five hours or so it takes for the spinal block to wear off.

Top tips for managing labour pain

Every woman experiences labour in a different way; it can be very painful for some, while others find it less so. Apart from medical relief, here are **gurgle's** tried and tested ways to help ease the pain.

DISTRACTION
Try taking a stroll along the hospital corridors (or if you are at home, around the house or garden) to take your mind off the pain. Reading, watching TV, or even something as simple as talking to your friends on the phone can all help too.

WATER
Water is a simple, soothing and relatively easy way to manage the pain. Most maternity units now have baths, showers and birthing pools for you to use during labour. If you are at home, getting into the bath or having a shower can help, but if your waters have broken already this is not advisable as infections can now reach your baby. (For more on the the benefits of water for labour and delivery, see pages 122–3.)

TENS MACHINE
Once you get the hang of it, a TENS machine can be very effective at reducing pain. Remember to hire one well before your due date and bear in mind that it can't be used in a birthing pool. (For more information, see page 119.)

HEAT
Applying something warm to your back – a hot-water bottle, heat pad or even a jumper warmed on the radiator – can help to ease labour pains and backache.

top tips

MASSAGE

Your birth partner doesn't need to have any training to do massage – you'll probably direct him or her! Having your lower back kneaded can help with any back pain and will ease some of the tension you may be feeling. A neck and shoulder massage is also a great way to relieve tension. Say what feels best and how hard or softly you want to be massaged.

HYPNOTHERAPY

Hypnotherapy can provide you with some very useful techniques for controlling pain and keeping you in a peaceful, positive frame of mind. (For more on this, see page 179; see also the section on HypnoBirthing, pages 124–5.)

BIRTHING BALL

Using your birthing ball throughout pregnancy can help strengthen your spine, helping avoid backache in labour. During labour, use your birthing ball to sit on, rock backwards and forwards on all fours, lie over and basically support your weight while you try different positions. Your maternity unit may have birthing balls already, so remember to ask your midwife at your next antenatal appointment. You can hire one if you are intending to have a home birth.

CONTROLLED BREATHING

Controlled breathing helps you to avoid tensing up while you are having a contraction, making it less painful. It also sends oxygen around your bloodstream and to your baby, which helps to make your muscles function more efficiently. (For how to breathe to help you through contractions, see pages 144–5.)

RESTING

Labour can be very long, but in between contractions, if you can rest, you should: your body needs all the energy it can get. Remember to stay well hydrated and try to eat small amounts of plain food like toast if possible.

top
tips

Assisted delivery – forceps or ventouse?

Your baby may need assistance to be delivered and this could be for a variety of reasons. You may be exhausted after pushing for a long time, or your baby may be making slow progress down the birth canal. Larger babies may require help, as may breech babies. If it is inadvisable for you to push for a prolonged period of time (if, for example, you suffer from heart disease), or if your baby is showing signs of distress, your doctor or midwife may also suggest a form of assisted delivery.

Ventouse delivery

A ventouse extraction uses suction to guide your baby out. Your legs will first be placed in supports or stirrups. Your doctor will place a device that looks a bit like a large cup on your baby's head and she will then be gently suctioned out as you push. She may have slight swelling on her head for about 24 hours after the birth, but this will soon return to normal.

Forceps delivery

Forceps are another option for assisted delivery if your baby needs to come out quickly. The end of the bed will be removed and your feet will be placed in stirrups. You will be given a catheter to drain your bladder. An episiotomy (a cut made in the vaginal opening) will be performed to create enough space to insert the forceps, which look a bit like metal salad tongs. Your doctor will fit them carefully around your baby's head and gently pull her out while you push. Some forceps can be used to turn your baby around if she is in an awkward position. Sometimes a baby born with the help of forceps can have two red marks on either side of her head, but these will disappear within the first week.

Mum's top tip

Don't worry that your baby's head will suffer if your carers decide to use forceps to help delivery. These are placed very gently over your baby's head and any bruising that results fades very quickly indeed. I'm actually glad that my carers opted for forceps, as if we had waited any longer I might have had to have a Caesarean delivery.

Episiotomy

Although once widely practised in childbirth, there is much debate about how beneficial episiotomies are. Some health professionals believe that tearing naturally in childbirth is better than having a surgical cut, as it heals more quickly and results in less postnatal pain and fewer problems with incontinence. Others believe that episiotomies heal better than tears.

An episiotomy is a procedure in which an incision is made in the perineum (the area between the vagina and anus) to enlarge the vaginal opening and make it easier for the baby's head to emerge. While routine episiotomies are no longer standard, there are reasons you may have to have one. If you have a large or breech baby, a forceps or ventouse delivery or your baby gets stuck in the birth canal, an episiotomy may be suggested.

The perineal area will be numbed with a local anaesthetic, and the cut will be made in one of two ways: a midline cut, which is a straight down cut towards the rectum, or a mediolateral cut, which is angled to one side, away from the rectum. The midline cut is easier to repair, and causes the mother less discomfort, but doctors favour the mediolateral cut because it is less likely to cause damage close to the rectum.

Medical staff these days try hard not to perform an episiotomy, unless it's really necessary, because of the painful healing process afterwards and the incontinence it can lead to. The good news is that evidence shows that, three months after giving birth, women who tear, those who don't and those who have episiotomies all have the same-strength pelvic-floor muscles.

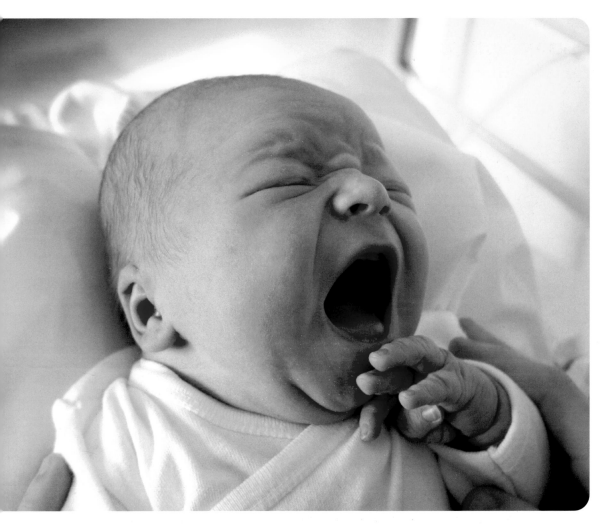

How painful is an episiotomy?

An episiotomy is performed in the last stages of labour and is unlikely to compete with the pain of a contraction. The area will be numbed while the procedure is performed and most women report that they didn't feel pain at all. In fact, a lot of women feel immediate relief, as in most cases it allows their baby to be born virtually straight away.

What about afterwards?

You will feel pain afterwards, once you have been stitched up and the anaesthetic has worn off, especially when you go to the loo. But there are a number of ways you can help yourself.

HOT AND COLD THERAPY
Place an ice pack on the stitches to reduce any swelling; if you are at home, you could use a packet of frozen peas. A warm bath can also soothe the area. Be careful to pat dry, rather than rub, the stitches afterwards.

WALKING AROUND
Although it may seem insane at first, the more you can walk around, the quicker you will heal.

AIR
Let the fresh air get to your stitches. Remove your knickers and lie on your bed with a towel under you to protect the sheets, and do this for at least ten minutes twice a day.

Avoiding an episiotomy

Many women swear by perineal massage, for 6–8 weeks before your due date, so that your perineum is used to being stretched before labour, reducing the need for an episiotomy.

Make sure your hands are clean and any jagged nails are trimmed beforehand. Apply olive oil or sweet almond oil (don't use any mineral-based oils, such as petroleum jelly) to the base of your vagina and your thumbs, then insert your thumbs into your vagina as far as the first knuckle. Now gently massage and stretch the tissues until you feel a slight burning sensation. Repeat the procedure every day. Of course, you can always ask your partner to do this for you, which might result in a lot more fun for both of you, and will certainly take your mind off episiotomies for a while!

It may also be possible to reduce your risk of needing an episiotomy by labouring in an upright position. Standing or squatting are good positions to try. A warm compress applied to the perineal area can also help.

Lots of women worry about episiotomies and how much they will hurt. It's true that they can be painful, especially in the first days after the delivery, but they also heal very quickly.

Mum's top tip

The best advice I was given after I had an episiotomy with my first son was how to lessen the stinging sensation when you pee. What you do is sit on the loo and gently dribble a cup of tepid water over your urethra as you urinate. The tepid water dilutes your pee and makes it less acidic, and so it stings less. After peeing, pat your bottom dry, from front to back, with a soft towel. You will start to heal rapidly and soon it won't sting at all when you pee.

Perineal tears

Although it does not always happen, it is common for your perineum (the area between your vagina and anus) to tear during the birth of your baby. There are different degrees of tearing:

Degrees of perineal tearing

FIRST-DEGREE TEAR
A first-degree tear is when there is minor tearing to the area around the entrance to the vagina. This will heal well, you'll feel little discomfort and in most cases will not need stitching.

SECOND-DEGREE TEAR
This is when the tear goes through the skin and the perineal muscles underneath. The anal sphincter muscles remain intact. Second-degree tears will need several stitches through the muscle and tissue in the perineal area. You will feel a certain amount of discomfort.

THIRD-DEGREE TEAR
This is where the anal sphincter muscles are torn, but the lining inside the rectum remains intact. These tears require careful stitching to repair.

FOURTH-DEGREE TEAR
This type of tear isn't common, occurring in only 1% of births. The anal sphincter is torn and the anal mucosa opened. You will need careful, skilled stitching to repair it.

Why might I tear?

While minor tearing is fairly common, third- and fourth-degree tears are not. You are more at risk from this type of tear if:

- You have had an assisted delivery: forceps or ventouse were used to help get your baby out (see pages 186–7)
- Your baby is bigger than normal
- Your baby is breech and is being delivered vaginally.

If I do tear, what will the treatment be?

Depending on the severity of the tear, it may require stitches. You will be given a local anaesthetic which will numb the area that needs to be stitched. Afterwards, it might give you some relief to apply a cold ice pack to the area or to request or accept additional medical pain relief. It might sting when you urinate for a while afterwards, but this will soon pass. You are advised to abstain from sex until you get the go-ahead from your GP, either at your six-week check-up or at a later check-up if you had a deep tear.

Having an episiotomy instead

Sometimes your midwife will suggest that you have an episiotomy instead of tearing, to make room for your baby to be born. Some people favour tearing because they feel that it is as nature intended. These days medical staff tend to perform episiotomies only if they are really needed (see pages 188–9). As with a natural tear, you will be stitched up following an episiotomy, and should heal very quickly. Bear in mind too that, as research shows, the strength of your pelvic-floor muscles will be the same three months after the birth, whether you had an episiotomy, tore naturally or didn't tear at all.

Avoiding tearing

Tearing is particularly common if this is your first baby. But there are steps you can take to help prevent it happening. Follow the advice given for avoiding an episiotomy (see pages 190–1).

Top tips for birthing partners

While watching your loved one in pain can be very hard to deal with, most men agree that seeing their baby enter the world is one of the most satisfying and exhilarating moments of their life. Whether you grab the video camera, cower in the corner or grunt along with your partner, you will want to offer the best support possible. Follow **gurgle's** top tips for getting ready for this special event.

PREPARE YOURSELF

Be as prepared as possible. It may be harrowing, and it will be tough, but the more you understand what is happening, the more in control you will both feel. Look through your partner's books on pregnancy and attend antenatal classes (see pages 110–11) with her, so you know exactly what to expect and when. Try not to be a know-it-all, however. While you can question anything you like, don't think you know more than the medical staff because you've read a few chapters on birth and labour. It's important that you work with the team, not against them.

STAY CALM

The last thing your partner needs is you having a panic attack when you see a bit of blood. Lots of people don't like needles or the sight of blood, of course, and if this is the case you may need to discuss this with your partner before the birth. Try to stay calm, even if all around you is chaos, so she can rely on someone constant and familiar next to her. It may be wise to stay at the 'top' rather than the 'business' end if you are feeling squeamish. That way you can keep in eye contact with your partner, giving lots of encouragement when things get tough.

top
tips

LOOK AFTER YOURSELF

It is OK to have a break. You may feel guilty taking time out when your partner has to grin and bear it, but it is important that you pace yourself. Labour can last for 12 hours plus, so make sure you get regular rests, don't forget to eat, and keep yourself well hydrated. Bring your own music to listen to, and stock up on newspapers, magazines and books. Don't forget that maternity wards are usually kept very warm for the sake of the babies, so you may need a couple of shirts to change into. Pack a T-shirt and shorts for the birth, as you will get hot and it can get messy, and make sure you have a change of clothes for afterwards. If you are finding it tough, have a quiet word with the midwife, who can relieve you while you get some fresh air.

BE HER ROCK

Support your partner in every way you can. Breathe together to help her establish a rhythm, be the back-rub guru – this can really help to ease the pain – and encourage her if she becomes disheartened or loses confidence. Help her to move into different positions such as standing, squatting, using the birthing ball, going on all fours. Don't take it to heart if she doesn't want to be held, or wants to be left alone. It is up to you to judge when to help and when to back off.

ENCOURAGE HER

Tell her she's doing well, that she will meet her baby very soon, that she is strong, that you are proud of her, that you love her, and that this will be over in no time. In the last stages of birth, tell her what you can see ('The baby's head is coming!') to give her a boost for the final push. Listen to her wishes: if she finds your encouragement annoying, back off a bit and give her some space.

top
tips

PROVIDE BACK UP

It is your responsibility to make sure the car is full of petrol, that you know where to park, you have change for the car park, your partner's labour bag and maternity notes are with you, and she has enough to eat, drink and distract her between contractions. She should only have to focus on the labour and birth, clearing all other worries from her mind. If you have other children, reassure her they are safe and happy, and that she will see them soon.

BE HER GO-BETWEEN

Help her to communicate what she wants, especially if she is in pain and cannot speak. There is no need to jump in and speak for her, but repeat the questions calmly between contractions. Familiarize yourself with her birth plan and what she wants the birth to be like, so you can let the midwives know if there are any changes.

Don't be afraid to ask questions if you don't understand what is happening. It might help to think of the word BRAIN when you are faced with a difficult decision, as the letters stand for important points to bear in mind:

B = What are the benefits?
R = What are the reasons for this?
A = Is there an alternative?
I = What do your partner's instincts tell you?
N = What would happen if we did nothing?

Happy birth day

If you go through this series of questions when you are faced with a tough decision – whether your partner should have a Caesarean section, for instance – it can help to rationalize the situation so that you can think more clearly.

BE HAPPY

Try to appear positive and happy about everything that is happening rather than looking horrified. Lots of women are worried about making noises during labour, or accidentally urinating or passing a stool. If she does, just laugh it off, give her a kiss and carry on with the encouragement.

BE FLEXIBLE

Birth plans change, babies come early or are overdue (and can interfere with big projects at work). Women in labour can be irrational and unpredictable. Help your partner deal with it when she does not get the natural water birth with whale music she had planned. Then, if it does happen, it will be an added bonus.

BE THERE

The most important thing you can do is be there for her. This really is a drop-everything situation. If you are focused, it will help her to be focused and in control, so don't sit chatting on your phone, or worrying about the meeting you are missing at work. Focus on your partner and give her encouragement, cuddles and lots of kisses. This is an important moment for you too. It is easy for birth partners to be forgotten in the hype that surrounds the birth, but this is your child too, and the birth should be a memorable and positive experience for you as well.

top tips

Your bundle of joy

Bonding after birth

Bonding is that intense attachment you feel when you look at your baby and want to hug and protect him, showering him with affection.

The ties you form with your baby are vital because they enable him to feel secure, confident and loved. Much of his emotional development depends on the closeness of his relationship with those around him from a very early age. It is important for bonding to happen straight away as, contrary to what you might think, babies are aware of their surroundings as soon as they are born.

HOLD HIM SKIN TO SKIN
Touch is essential, especially skin-to-skin contact. If your baby is premature, you will be encouraged to hold him naked next to your chest, or touch and stroke him as much as possible if he is in an incubator. Your body will keep him warm and he will develop a sense of security, familiarity and comfort from being close to you. He will also get used to how you feel and smell.

KEEP UP THE EYE CONTACT
Use as much eye contact as possible. Remember your baby can only see objects up to 20–30cm (8–12in) from him, so bring your face close to his, look at him and smile. Babies have an innate ability to recognize human faces and he will love looking at yours. He may try to imitate your facial expressions – try sticking your tongue out to see if he can copy you. Although his first words won't appear for some months yet, he may even try a few little noises, his first attempts at communication.

TALK IN A SOOTHING VOICE
Talk to him in a soothing voice, telling him how much you love him, that you are here for him. It may seem silly talking to someone who does not understand you or respond, but he is taking it all in and it will help him communicate and socialize.

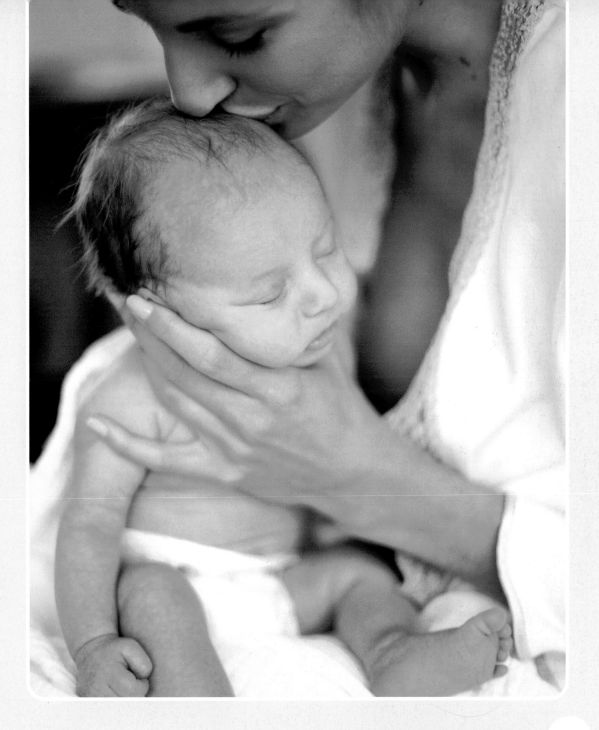

Dads: bonding with your new baby

In those first weeks after your baby arrives, your partner may start to feel excluded when it comes to caring for his new child. Watching the bond between mother and baby grow, he may feel a sense of rejection or helplessness – how can he possibly start forging a bond with a child who seems so utterly dependent on mum?

Many first-time dads assume that women 'instinctively' know how to look after babies, but this isn't always the case. For a woman who has never had younger siblings, her own baby may well be her first experience of caring for a young child. She's likely to be as clueless as you are about the practicalities of looking after your baby, so share the care and find out together.

GET INVOLVED FROM DAY ONE
Do your share of nappy changes, baths and bedtimes right from the start so that you get to know your baby and feel confident looking after her on your own.

HELP WITH FEEDS
Unless your baby is being exclusively breastfed, you can do some of her feeds yourself. If she is breastfed, don't forget that once breastfeeding is established, your partner can express some of her breast milk and you can feed it to your baby from a bottle, if you wish.

TAKE THE TIME TO READ UP
Your partner has mostly likely been devouring books about babies for months, so why not look through one yourself? Knowing about labour and birth and how to care for your baby will enable you to feel more confident about helping out.

TAKE YOUR BABY WITH YOU

What better way to get to know your baby than to take her with you as you go about some daily chores? Strap her in the sling and get out in the garden or take her shopping with you. Even if your baby is exclusively breastfed, a 20-minute stroll together will give you valuable bonding time as well as a small break for mum.

DON'T BE A DEAF DAD

Be prepared to sometimes be the one who gets up at night to give your baby a feed, wind her and change her nappy, or maybe just soothe her back to sleep.

MAKE SPECIAL TIME TOGETHER

Due to work pressure, many dads see far less of their new babies than they would like so make an effort to get involved when you are around, such as at weekends or during holidays. Have a 'dad and baby' time at weekends. This can be your special time to do things together, such as going for walks or taking swimming lessons – giving mum a well-deserved break.

LEARN HOW TO SOOTHE YOUR BABY

Don't fall into the trap of simply handing your baby back to your partner when she cries. Dads can be just as good as mums at soothing babies, and learning what is upsetting your baby and how to solve it is the first form of communication between children and parents.

Mum's top tip

When I had a Caesarean, I was so glad that my husband was with me. As soon as our son arrived, the surgeon handed him to my husband. The midwife encouraged him to hold the baby against his bare chest in those first few moments. Both father and son looked so calm. I'll never forget those enquiring eyes, looking at his dad. That bonding from the first moment is so special – make the most of it.

Becoming parents

Although having a baby is a very exciting time, it can also be a challenging one. Suddenly, you and your partner are making the transition from being a couple to becoming a family. Although you both have so much to look forward to together, you won't be able to enjoy the quality time with each other that you're used to. Spontaneous weekend breaks and those long weekend lie-ins are a thing of the past now. The sacrifice will be worth it, but it does take some getting used to.

When your baby arrives, you won't feel like leaving him for a while, but you do need to make time for yourselves. It's normal to go off sex when you've recently given birth, as suddenly you don't seem to have either the time or the inclination to be sensual and physical. However, it's important to remember that intimacy is a vital part of any relationship as it helps to make you feel closer to your partner. This isn't to say that you should rush things, however. It's probably best to wait a few weeks after you've given birth before you resume having sex, as your body needs time to recover. Wait until your GP has given you the all-clear.

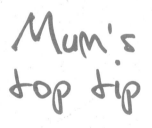

Every relationship is different – there's no such thing as a perfect one! My advice is don't set yourself high ideals which you constantly try to live up to, but give yourselves a bit of a break. If you and your partner do snap at each other, don't beat yourself up about it. When your bundle of joy arrives, he or she will alter everything and, if you let it, it will change your life for the better.

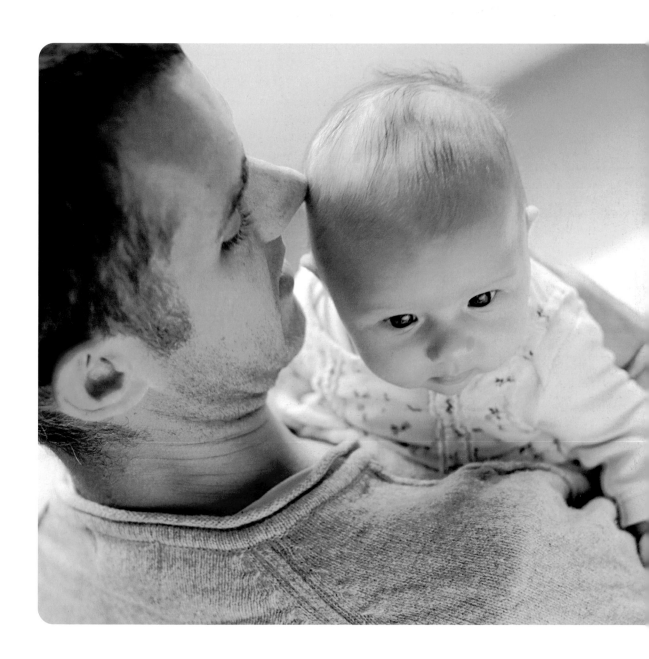

How should I hold my newborn baby?

It is perfectly safe for friends and relatives to hold your baby, but make sure they are holding her correctly. Newborn babies have very little head control and their heads will loll to one side if they are not supported. If yours is picked up awkwardly and is uncomfortable, rest assured she will let the world know with a yelp and a scream.

1 Cradle your baby in your arms. This is often referred to as the 'cradle hold' and is very comfortable for the baby.

3 Hold your baby against your shoulder with her head turned to the side and her back supported by your hand.

2 Newborn babies love to be held across your arm. Lay her on her front, with her head on your wrist and her legs dangling either side of your elbow. Your forearm is basically supporting her body and she resembles a lion cub lying astride a branch.

 For the **gurgle** video on **How to hold your newborn** and **Bathing your newborn** go to **gurgle.com** and click on **Videos**

Important points to remember about holding a newborn

1 Make sure that all visitors have washed their hands.

2 Don't let young children hold your baby without supervision.

3 If your baby is being passed from relative to relative, don't be afraid to take her back for a bit of quiet mummy time. Your baby can get overstimulated and anxious if she is passed among unfamiliar faces, so give her a break after a while.

Anatomy of a newborn

- The soft spots on your baby's head are known as fontanelles and sometimes you can see them pulsating. Try not to press them. (These will have closed up by the time your child is about 18 months.)

- Your baby's eyes may look puffy and closed, but they will open in time. Nearly all babies are born with blue or blue-grey eyes, but permanent eye coloration will develop over the first few months.

- Her fingers will be curled up in little balls.

- Her umbilical cord will have been cut and clamped and there will be a stump which will fall off after a few days.

- Her limbs are curled up, as they were in your womb, but they will uncurl over time.

- Babies' genitals are usually swollen and enlarged after delivery and for a few days afterwards because of hormones passed to them from your body.

- Her hands and feet may be covered in dry, peeling skin for a while as her skin adjusts to conditions outside the womb.

Tests and checks for newborn babies

Immediately after your baby is born, a series of checks will be performed on him, just to make sure everything is working properly.

Apgar test

The Apgar test is performed at one- and five-minute intervals after your baby has been delivered. Named after Dr Virginia Apgar, who developed the test, the individual letters each stand for a particular feature the medical team will be checking.

'A' FOR APPEARANCE
Your baby's skin colour will be checked to see if it is a healthy shade; if not, his skin may be gently rubbed to help the blood start circulating.

'P' FOR PULSE
A good pulse reading is normally anything over 100.

'G' FOR GRIMACE
Your baby's cries, coughs or sneezes represent good responses to external stimulation.

'A' FOR ACTIVITY
The more your baby moves around the better.

'R' FOR RESPIRATION
A good healthy cry means your baby has clear airways and his lungs are working.

Once the Apgar test has been carried out, your baby's fingers and toes, spine, anus and facial features will be checked, and his head and length measured. His hips will also be checked. Breech babies may need extra checks on their hips because of the position they occupied in the womb, so ask your midwife or health visitor about this if you were not offered one at the hospital.

Vitamin K

All babies are born with lower levels of vitamin K – vital for the blood-clotting process – than adults. A small number of babies (about 1 in 10,000) suffer from what is known as 'vitamin K deficiency bleeding' or VKDB, a rare condition that usually emerges in the first week of life, in which a baby's blood may not clot properly. This can result in bleeding in the brain, which in turn can lead to brain damage or, in some cases, death. This is why a vitamin K injection is offered to newborns, usually within the first hour after they are born.

CONCERNS ABOUT VITAMIN K

Some people have concerns about the vitamin K injection because of research carried out in the early 1990s that suggested giving the injection to babies may also be linked to childhood leukaemia (a blood cancer). Since the original study, several other studies have been conducted in the UK, Germany, Scotland and the US, but none have found conclusive evidence that the vitamin K injection is linked to childhood leukaemia. In addition, there is no evidence to suggest that the oral dose of Vitamin K has any links to childhood cancer.

WHICH BABIES ARE AT RISK OF VKDB?

Because of the low levels of vitamin K in breast milk during the early postnatal period, babies who are exclusively breastfed are slightly more at risk. VKDB is also more common in babies who are premature, or who have had a complicated delivery (such as breech, or delivery by ventouse or forceps).

It is important to remember that breast milk is the best food for babies, so even though the VKDB risks are higher in breastfed infants, this should not put you off breastfeeding. The benefits of breastfeeding outweigh all other factors, giving your baby the best possible start in life.

WHY IS VITAMIN K GIVEN TO ALL BABIES?

In about one in three cases, VKDB occurs with no prior warning to babies who are not in a high-risk category. For this reason, vitamin K is offered to all newborns. As parents, you have the right to choose whether your baby receives this injection, but your midwife may recommend he has it, depending on the circumstances.

HOW IS VITAMIN K GIVEN?

Vitamin K is usually administered by injection, in a single dose, but it can also be given orally. The oral dose has to be given once after birth and again a month later. All hospitals have different protocols about when and how vitamin K is given, so ask your midwife at your next appointment which procedure she follows. If you are concerned about the vitamin K injection, talk to your GP or midwife before your baby is born.

Mum's top tip

Keep your baby's identity bracelet in a safe place once you're home from hospital. The bracelets are fitted once all the newborn tests are completed. Your baby will grow quickly and when he's old enough to understand, he'll be amazed to think how tiny his wrists and ankles once were.

Your bundle of joy

Weight

Your baby will be weighed immediately after delivery, and will then be weighed regularly in the hospital, or by your midwife if you have a home birth. Your health visitor will visit you once you have brought your baby home, to check his weight and that he and you are doing well. Babies usually lose a bit of weight straight after they are born – until they master feeding – but they should regain it by the time they are a week old.

Heel prick test

Some babies need to have a test where blood is taken from their heel, to check thyroid function and also for a rare disorder called phenylketonuria (causing problems with brain development). Your baby's heel will be pricked and a small amount of blood taken for the test. This should not hurt your baby.

Keeping fully informed

When each test is being performed on your newborn, make sure you ask what the test is and why your baby needs it. It is your right to know what is happening to your baby, and medical staff will be happy to answer any questions.

The first nappies

Your baby's first stool is called meconium and is black- or green-looking, mostly made up of digested mucus. Meconium is normally passed within the first 24 hours. Your baby's next bowel movement can be up to two days later, especially if you are breastfeeding. After your baby has passed meconium, the next stools will probably be greenish-brown, then a yellowy colour. The stools of bottlefed babies will be a little more solid, but will also be a similar yellowy shade.

Your baby should have several wet nappies a day, as he's not able to hold urine for long. If his urine is stained pink or red, don't worry; this is normal for a newborn and will soon return to a clear colour.

Vaginal discharge

Don't worry if your newborn baby girl has a small amount of clear or white vaginal discharge in her nappy, or even a bit of vaginal bleeding. This is perfectly normal and is due to the hormones in your body being passed to your baby. Show your midwife or doctor if you are worried.

Tests for sight and hearing

Newborn babies cannot see very far, no further than about 20–30cm (8–12in). Reassuringly for the mother, this is approximately the same distance between you and your baby when you are holding her at your breast, so she will stare at you intently while you hold her. Don't be alarmed if your baby looks cross-eyed at first; this is just her eye muscles adjusting, and will stop after a few weeks.

Your baby's hearing is well developed when she is born and she may turn to look if she hears a loud sound or towards a voice she recognizes (mummy or daddy). Some babies are offered hearing tests in the hospital, but this depends on the hospital's newborn-screening programme. Ask your health visitor what the procedures are in your area if your baby did not receive a hearing test in hospital; most babies are offered one at around six to eight months.

Six-week check-up

After six weeks, you and your baby will be checked by your GP to make sure that you are healing well from the birth, that feeding is going well and that your baby is steadily gaining in weight. The GP will also perform a physical examination on you to check that your uterus has moved back to its pre-pregnancy position. It might be a good idea to write down any concerns or questions you have during these early weeks so you can discuss them with your GP at the six-week check-up.

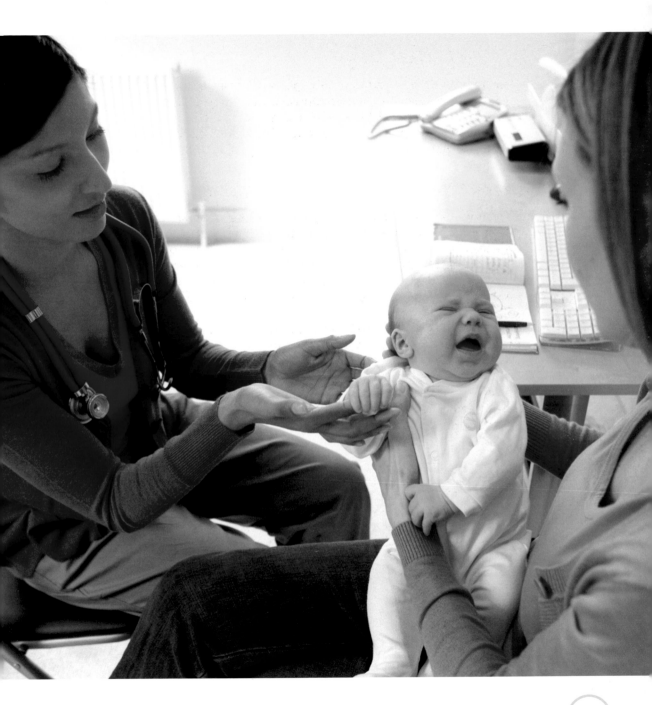

What will my newborn do?

Returning home with your precious new bundle is a joyful experience but it can also seem a daunting one at first. Bear in mind that your newborn baby's needs are very simple – to eat, sleep and be loved – and you'll soon find you adapt to your new life together.

SLEEP

Newborn babies have one important thing to do – grow bigger. For this they need plenty of sleep. Newborns sleep around 16 hours in every 24, and it may seem at first that not many of these are actually at night! They sleep in two-, three- or four-hour bursts until they are old enough to go for longer between feeds, and can handle a sleep routine. In the beginning, there is no need to implement a routine. Your baby will sleep when she needs to. This is an important part of her growing process, so try not to be strict with her just yet.

As a new parent, the lack of sleep and being woken up repeatedly at three, four, and five in the morning will make you irritable, tired and grumpy. Try to catch up on sleep during the day, when your baby is napping, and persuade your partner, parents or a friend to come and mind your baby occasionally so that you can have a welcome lie-in.

EAT

Apart from sleep, the chief activity of a newborn is to eat. Whether you are bottle- or breastfeeding, your baby will probably get hungry roughly every three hours, depending on her size and appetite. Newborn babies cannot hold much food as their stomachs are still very small; this is why they poo constantly. If you think all your baby does is eat, rest assured that, in time, her eating patterns will settle down and you won't always feel like you're doing non-stop, back-to-back feeding.

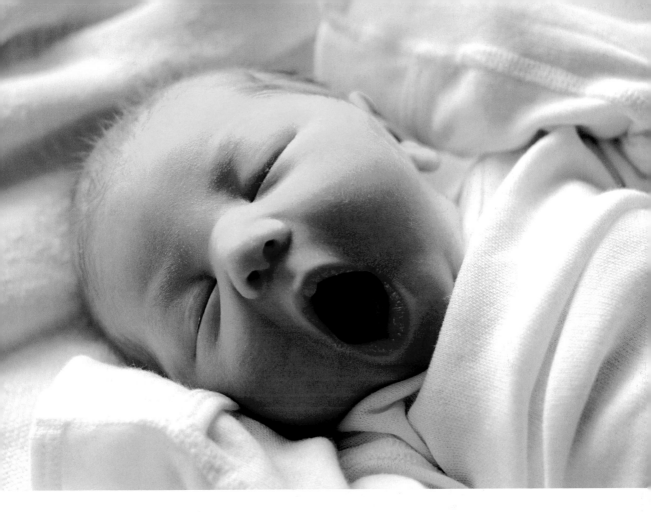

CRY

Newborn babies have only one way of communicating what they want – that is, to cry. The heartbreaking sound has new parents around the world literally pulling their hair out trying to work out what their baby needs. The good thing about newborn babies is that there are only a handful of things that actually make them cry, so it may be a simple process of elimination until you find out which it is. Newborns cry between one and three hours a day, but by the time your baby is a few weeks old, you will probably be able to distinguish which cry means she's hungry and which one means she needs a cuddle.

What will my newborn do?

Resources

AIMS
Association for Improvements in Maternity
Services
For help obtaining maternity care
0870 765 1433
www.aims.org.uk

ARC (Antenatal Results and Choices)
Advice on antenatal tests and results
0207 631 0285
www.arc-uk.org

Association of Postnatal Illness
Offering support to mums suffering from
postnatal illness
0207 386 0868
www.apni.org

Birth Works
Birthpool advice and hire
020 8244 0793
www.birthworks.co.uk

BLISS Baby Life Support System
Support for parents of special care babies
0500 618 140
www.bliss.org

Doula UK
The non-profit organization for doulas
in the UK
0871 433 3103
www.doula.org.uk

Down's Syndrome Association
Helps people with Down's syndrome to live
full lives
0845 230 0372
www.downs-syndrome.org.uk

Ectopic Pregnancy Trust
Providing a range of support and
information on ectopic pregnancies
020 7733 2653
www.ectopic.org.uk

**The Foundation for the Study of Infant
Deaths**
The UK's leading baby charity working to
prevent sudden deaths and promote health
020 7233 2090
www.sids.org.uk

Gingerbread
Local self-help groups for single parents and
their children
0800 018 4318
www.gingerbread.org.uk

HypnoBirthing UK
Self-hypnosis and breathing techniques for
labour and birth
www.HypnoBirthing.co.uk

Independent Midwives Association
Fully-qualified midwives who practice
outside the NHS
0845 4600 105
www.independentmidwives.org.uk

MAMA (Meet-A-Mum Association)
Offering invaluable sympathy and support
from other mums
0845 120 3746
www.mama.co.uk

Maternity Alliance
Promotes wellbeing of pregnant women,
new parents and babies
www.maternityalliance.org.uk

The Miscarriage Association
Offering information about miscarriages,
comfort and support
01924 200799
www.miscarriageassociation.org.uk

NCT (National Childbirth Trust)
Offering guidance on pregnancy, parenting
and birth
0870 444 8708
www.nct.org.uk

NHS Direct
National helpline offering medical
guidance and health information
0845 4647
www.nhsdirect.org.uk

Parentline Plus
Information and support for families
0808 800 2222
www.parentlineplus.org.uk

QUIT
Practical help to stop smoking
0800 00 22 00
www.quit.org.uk

Stillbirth and Neonatal death (SANDS)
Offering support to anyone affected by the
death of a baby
0207 436 5881
www.uk-sands.org

**TAMBA (Twins and Multiple Births
Association)**
Provides support for families of twins,
triplets and more
0800 138 0509
www.tamba.org.uk

**High street shops that sell
maternity ranges**
Dorothy Perkins www.dorothyperkins.com
H&M www.hm.com
Next www.next.co.uk
M&S www.marksandspencer.com
Mamas & Papas
www.mamasandpapas.co.uk
Mothercare www.mothercare.com
Topshop Maternity www.topshop.co.uk
Zara www.zara.com

Index

Acknowledgements

We would like to thank the **gurgle** experts' panel for their invaluable help in putting together this book. They are: Thirza Ashelford, MA FRSA Principal, Norland College; Alison Brown, registered midwife and registered general nurse; Dr Dorothy Einon, BSc, Phd, child development expert; Fiona Ford, MSc and dietician, co-director of the Centre for Pregnancy Nutrition, University of Sheffield; Eileen Hayes, MSc, BSc, parenting expert, writer and broadcaster; Dr Rob Hicks, MBBS, DRCOG, MRCGP, writer and broadcaster. The publishers would also like to thank Elizabeth Day, parenting consultant.

Text credits

Professor Jérôme Lejeune, *Discovery of the extra chromosome in Trisomy 21* (1959); Dr. Virginia Apgar, *A proposal for a new method of evaluation of the newborn infant* (1953).

Picture credits

All images, other than those listed below, have been provided by **gurgle.com**

16 Kate Mitchell/zefa/Corbis; 23 Gelpi; 32 gingging; 37 Ephraim Ben-Shimon/Corbis; 51 Magdalena Szachowska; 55 Leah-Anne Thompson; 57 Paul Mitchell/Mother & Baby Picture Library; 59 Ariel Skelley/Corbis; 69 Anna Dzondzua; 73 iofoto; 85 Juice Images/Corbis; 92 Zsolt Nyulaszi; 99 Nick Stubbs; 112 Leah-Anne Thompson; 120 Petro Feketa; 127 Zholobov Vadim; 133 Leah-Anne Thompson; 142 Mikko Pitkänen; 163 Ian Hooton/Mother & Baby Picture Library; 168 Stanislav Popov; 177 Supri Suharjoto; 181 Monkey Business Images; 189 Stephen Morris; 201 Ian Hooton/Mother & Baby Picture Library; 205 Bubbles Photolibrary/Alamy; 213 Ian Hooton/Mother & Baby Picture Library; 215 Vivid Pixels.